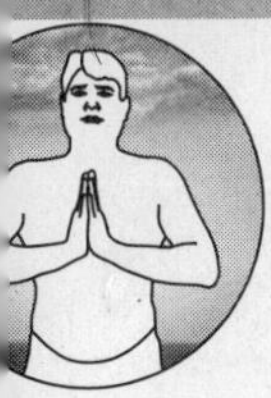

SURYA NAMASKAR

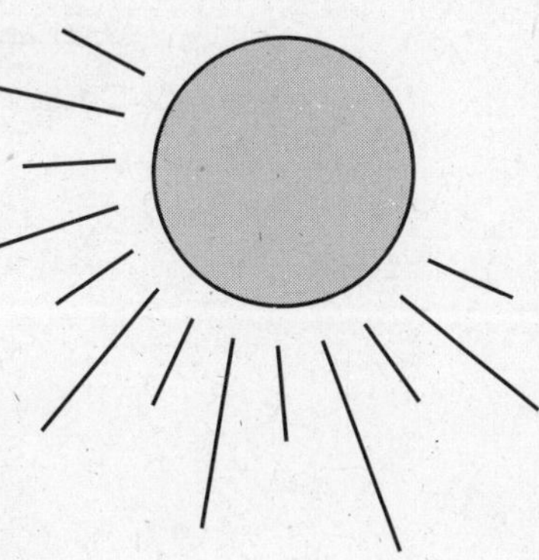

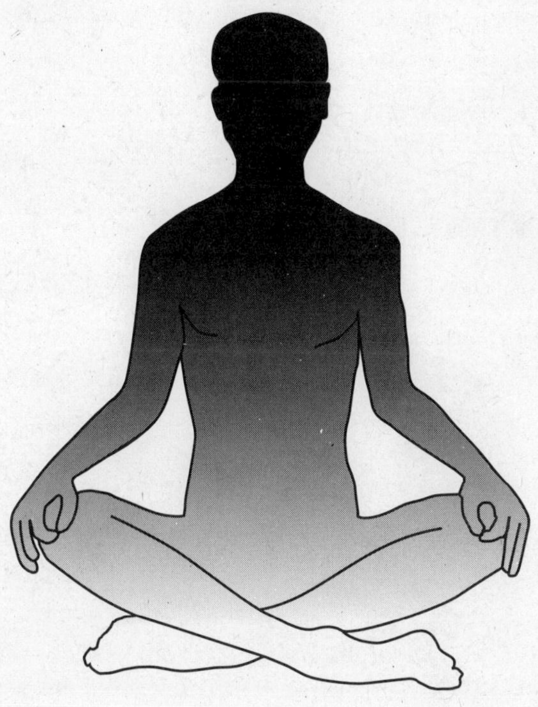

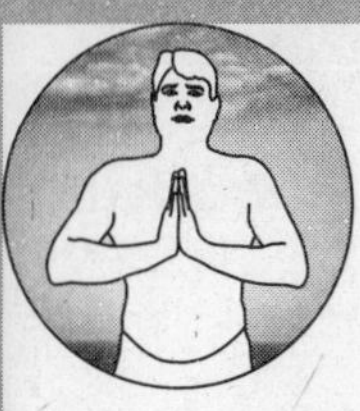

Surya Namaskar

SURYA NAMASKAR

Dr. Rajiv Rastogi
Dr. Sanjeev Rastogi

Ocean Books Pvt. Ltd.
ISO 9001:2000 Publishers

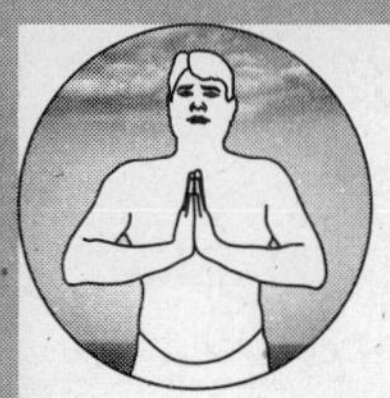

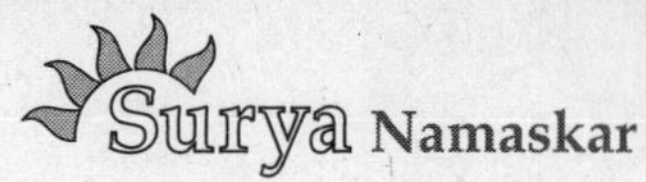

Published by
Ocean Books (P) Ltd.
4/19 Asaf Ali Road,
New Delhi-110 002 (INDIA)
e-mail: info@oceanbooks.in

ISBN 978-81-8430-349-0
Surya Namaskar
by Dr. Rajiv Rastogi & Dr. Sanjeev Rastogi

Edition
2024

Price
₹ 250.00 (Rupees Two Hundred Fifty only)

Design & Illustration by
Kalakriti Production, New Delhi

Printed at
Narula Printers, Delhi

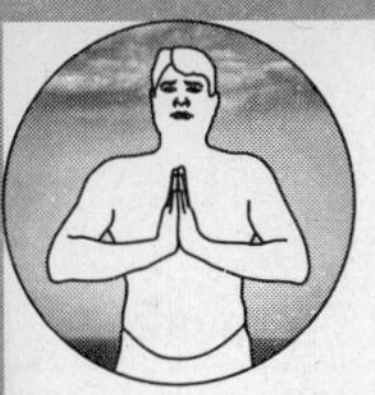

Contents

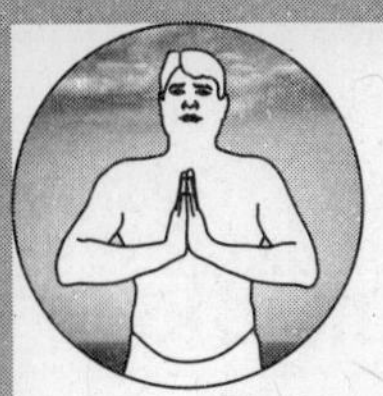

Preface

Surya Namaskar is a wonder gift from the Divine to us. The sun is the divine source of energy; hence the regular practice of Surya Namaskar not only enhances the functioning of our system but also revives and rejuvenates our whole body at the same time.

Yoga and Naturopathy are global sciences now. Thousands of people practise them regularly and include these sciences in their lifestyles to prevent various disorders. These practices are extremely effective, simple and easy to follow and produce amazing results. Anyone can learn and adopt them.

Earlier I wrote an article on 'Sun Salutation' titled *Surya Namaskar – Swasthya ka Aadhar* in Hindi which was published in the *Swagat* magazine of Indian Airlines. The article was appreciated and well received. Since my childhood, Surya Namaskar has attracted me a lot and I use to practise it, but not regularly. During a course on Naturopathy and Yoga, I got familiar with Surya Namaskar and its benefits. Since then it has been on my mind to write a book on the benefits of Surya Namaskar, the secret of complete health for the common man. But owing to some reasons, it was not possible to do so.

Later, working in a research organisation, I felt that a book on *Surya Namaskar* should be research-oriented but at the same time, in a simple and understandable language. The description should be palatable to researchers and the common man and should cover all the aspects of Surya Namaskar.

Ultimately, a manuscript was prepared after deep consultation with Dr. Sanjeev Rastogi, my younger brother and a leading Ayurvedic practitioner who is well-known for his new thoughts in medical practice and in writing books.

Now the book is in your hands. Though we have tried our level best to write the book in a way more convincing and useful for the common man, we believe that the readers of the book are the best judges. We hope that the book will be welcomed by people from all walks of life and will enhance the practice of Surya Namaskar for gaining perfect health.

New Delhi,
Teachers' Day, September 5, 2006

Authors

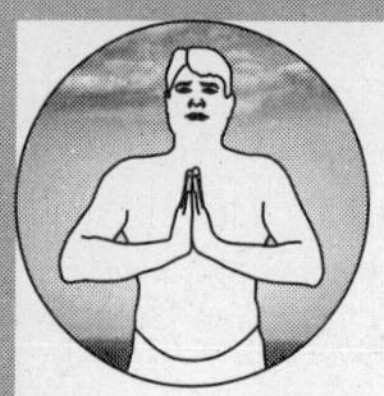

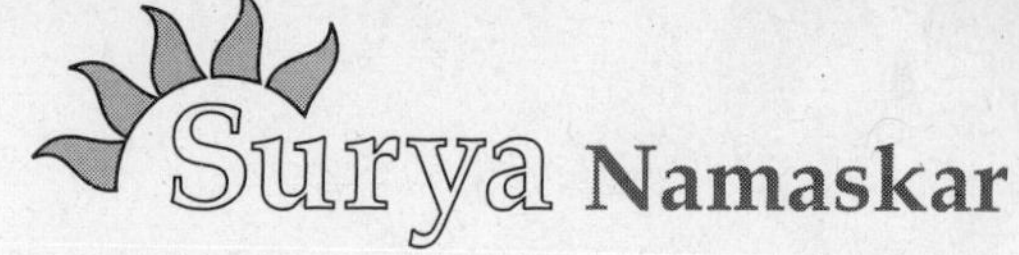

One who is the provider of vitality, life and energy to the whole universe, who is also worshipped by the gods, what else can be worshipped by the offerings?

Hiranyagarbha Sukta 2

Rigveda 10.121

The rising sun is the eliminator of death

Atharvaveda 17.1.30

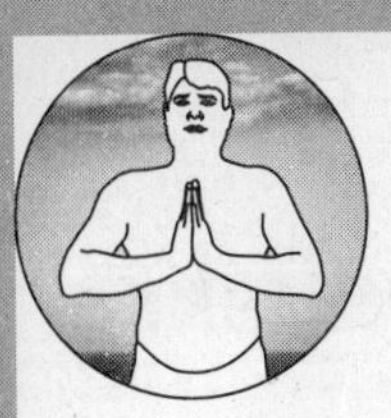

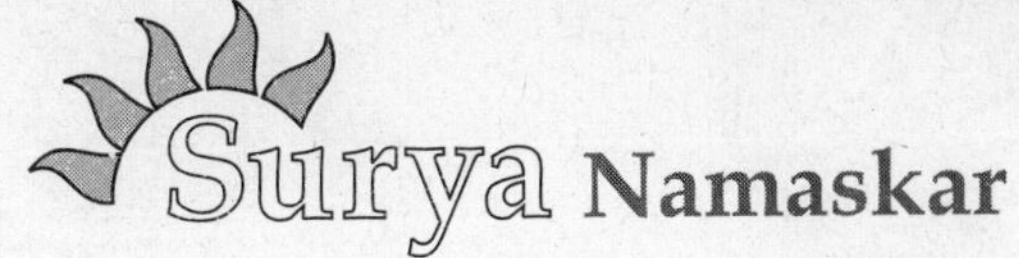

1. Introduction

As one of the most conspicuous and powerful subjects in the physical world, the sun has naturally attracted the attention and received homage from many races and civilisations that have personified and worshipped it as a god. Of these civilisations, sun worship was most practised by Vedic Indians, Persians, Greeks and Romans. Surprisingly, these were the most advanced civilisations of their times and they had associated many rituals beautifully into sun-worship which were basically meant to thank the unconditional support of the sun, essential for the sustenance of life in the universe. However, there were plenty of unseen rewards which came back as return gifts from the sun while performing the rituals for it and this might be the actual idea behind the blending of certain rituals with religious thoughts so that everyone for one reason or the other can be benefitted to the maximum by the treasures of nature. History is full of legends and monuments associated with this belief of the sun as the ultimate giver of life and healer. Famous among them are

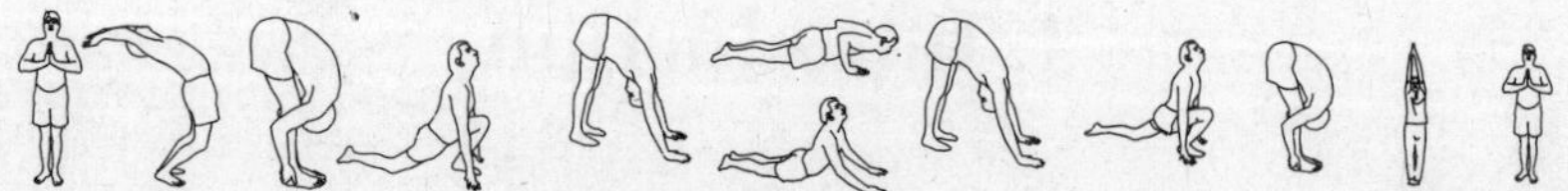

the Sun Temple at Konark and at Modhera in India and The Ri Tan (Ri = sun, Tan = temple) at Beijing, China.

The Sun Temple of Konark stands on a deserted stretch on the coast of Orissa, overlooking the Bay of Bengal. For centuries, this once lofty building was used by sailors navigating the shore. They called it the "Black Pagoda" to distinguish it from the "White Pagoda", the famous Jagannatha Temple. No one really knows why the Sun Temple was erected here, but there are many legends to account for its appearance. The most popular concerns Samba, the son of Lord Krishna. Samba was inordinately proud of his beauty. So proud that he once made the mistake of ridiculing a celebrated sage, Narada, who was always mischievous, Narada decided to have his revenge on the arrogant boy. He managed to lure the unsuspecting Samba to the pool where his stepmothers, the luscious consorts of Krishna, were bathing in joyful abandon. When Krishna heard that his son had become a peeping Tom, he was furious and cursed him with leprosy. Realising later

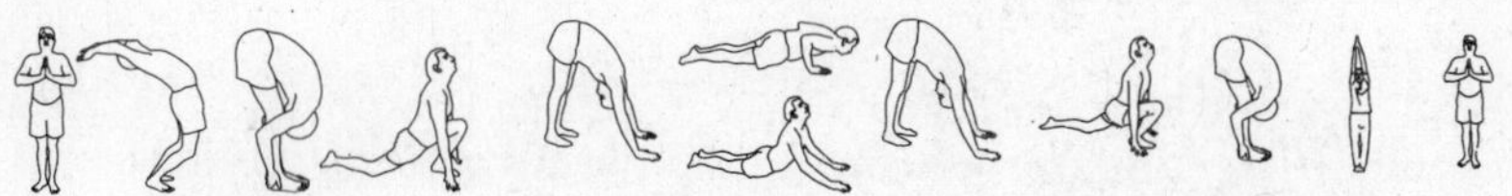

that the innocent boy had been tricked by Narada's cunning, Krishna was mortified.

But he could not revoke his curse; all he could do was advise his son to worship the Sun God, Surya, healer of all. But he could not revoke his curse; all he could do was advise his son to worship the Sun God, Surya, healer of all diseases, and hope for a cure.

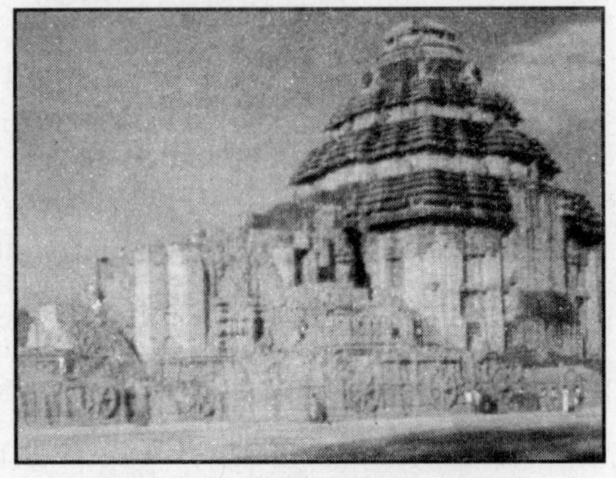

Sun Temple at Konark

After twelve years of penance and worship, Samba was at last instructed by Surya to go and bathe in the sea at Konark. He did so and was cured of his awful affliction. Samba was so delighted that he decided there and then to erect a Surya Temple on the spot. It was called Konark, "Place of the Sun," from which it derives its modern name.

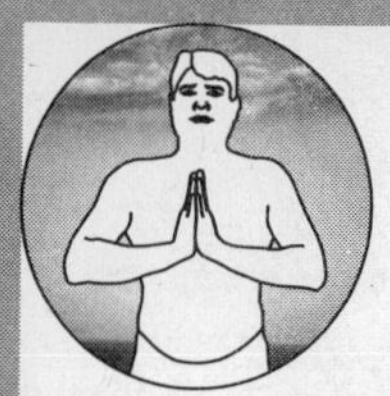

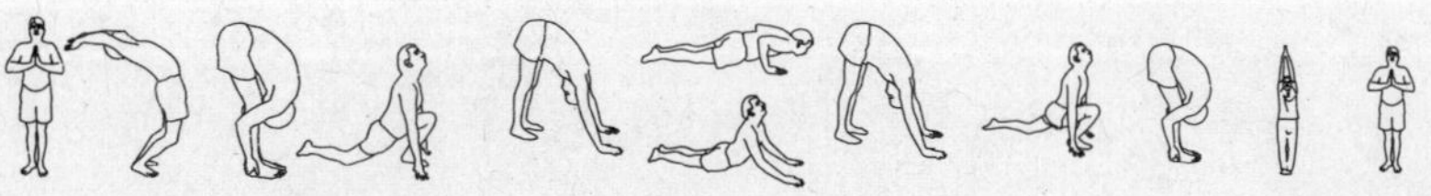

The temple was actually built by a king of the medieval Ganga dynasty, Narasingha Deva. The king was popularly known as Langulia, "the one with a tail." It is possible that he built the temple as a supplication to Surya to remove a spinal swelling of some sort.

The temple was conceived as a massive chariot lying on an east-west axis, in which the Sun God, Surya, was pulled across the sky. Each day his journey brought life and light back to earth and his procession was a continual rejoicing. The chariot had twenty-four wheels, and was pulled by seven horses, representing the seven days of the week and the seven sages who govern the constellations. Sun-worship is central to India. The standard daily prayer of the Brahmins is the *Gayatri*, addressed to the sun, and on an esoteric level, the sun symbolises the Divine Self within.

Ri Tan

Situated in Beijing, China, the Ri Tan symbolises the unity of cultural ideas in different civilisations that have

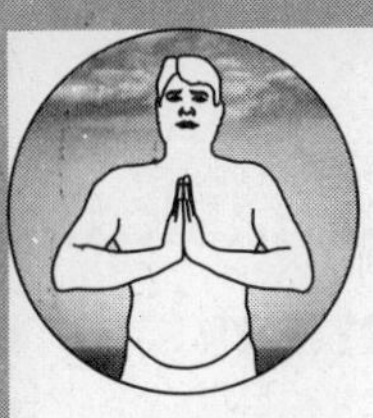

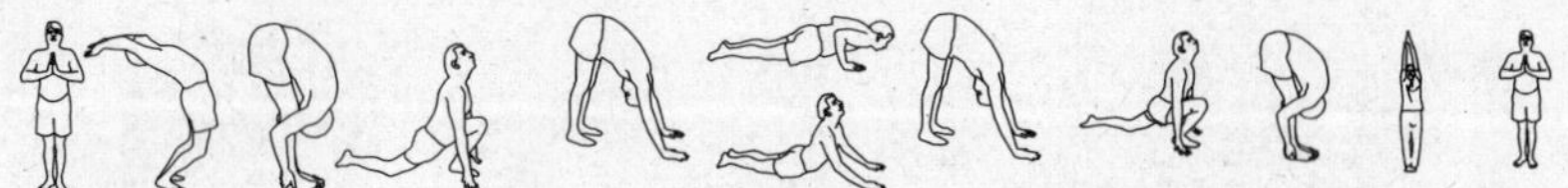

learned a lot from nature and in respect for the rewards given by nature, they have started praying to them as gods. The Temple of the Sun (Ri Tan) served as an altar where the emperor conducted annual rites. Built in 1530, Ri Tan now has a pleasant park and is situated in the east of the city. The other imperial altars are located in similar city parks, roughly marking the five points of the Chinese compass. To the north is Di Tan Gongyuan (Temple of the Earth), to the west is Yue Tan Gongyuan (Temple of the Moon); the much grander Tian Tan Gongyuan (Temple of Heaven) marks the southern point. She Ji Tan (Altar of Land and Grain) in Zhongshan Gongyuan, south-west of the Forbidden City, pre-dates them all by several centuries, and marks that peculiarly Chinese compass point, the centre.

Modhera is also famous for the Sun Temple, which is one of the finest examples of Indian temple architecture of its period. Built in 1026 AD, the temple is dedicated to the Sun God, Surya and stands high on a plinth overlooking a

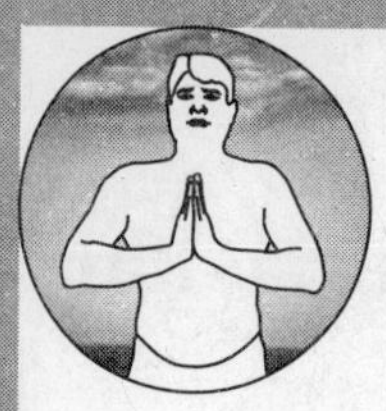

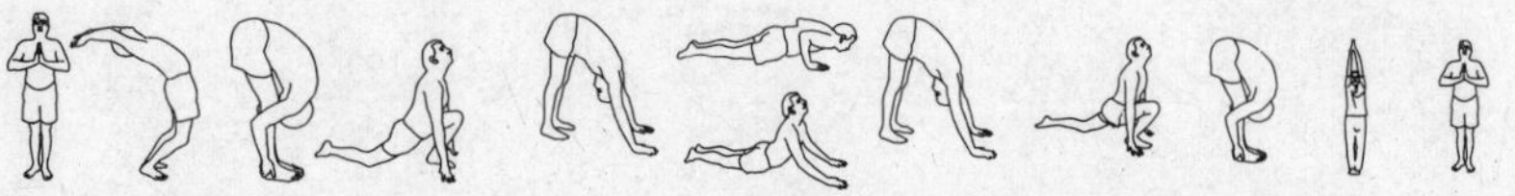

deep stone-stepped tank. As in the Sun Temple at Konark, this temple was so designed that the rays of the sun would fall on the image of Surya at the time of the equinoxes. Ruins of the Sun Temple at Modhera in Gujarat show considerable Magha influence. The walls of the temple have representations of the Sun God wearing a peculiar West Asian belt and boots as in the Sun Temple at Gaya. Mention must also be made of the huge tank in front of the temple with its multitude of images.

Built in 1026 during the reign of King Bhimdev I of the Solanki dynasty, the temple is dedicated to the Sun God. Destroyed by Mahmud of Ghazni, the Modhera temple still retains enough of its structure to convey the grandeur of its conception. Every inch of the edifice, both inside and outside, is magnificently carved with gods and goddesses, birds, beasts and flowers. The inner sanctum, which housed the presiding deity, faces east and was so designed that during the solar equinox, the first rays of the rising sun lit up the image of Surya.

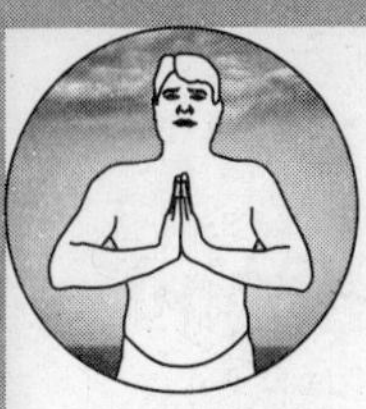

Surya Namaskar

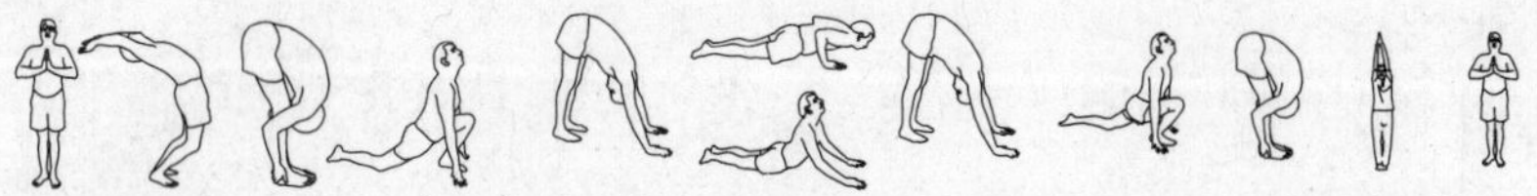

From the time of the Vedas to medieval times, sun-worship has been in existence in some form or the other. Every form of culture and every civilisation has taken note of this and has incorporated it in some way into their routine rituals to get the benefit from the sun. The sun is the representative of *agni* in the body. This is the embodiment of the theory that the body and nature have similar compositions and thus any deficiency or excess can truly be managed through nature alone. The sun has the property to dry water through evaporation. This can similarly be used to reduce the water principle of the living body called *kapha*. For the diseases caused by excess of *kapha* exposure to the sun is a good medicine.

Current day naturopaths have duly used this phenomenon and have advocated sitting under the sun for various clinical conditions. Another form of sun therapy is chromo therapy which uses the different colour components of sunrays to treat diseases.

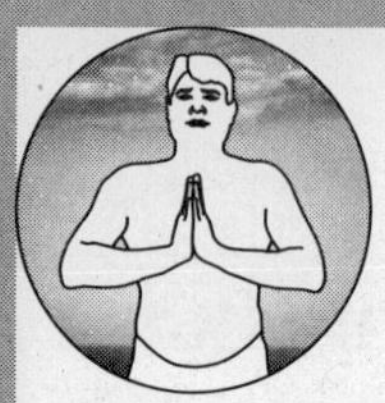

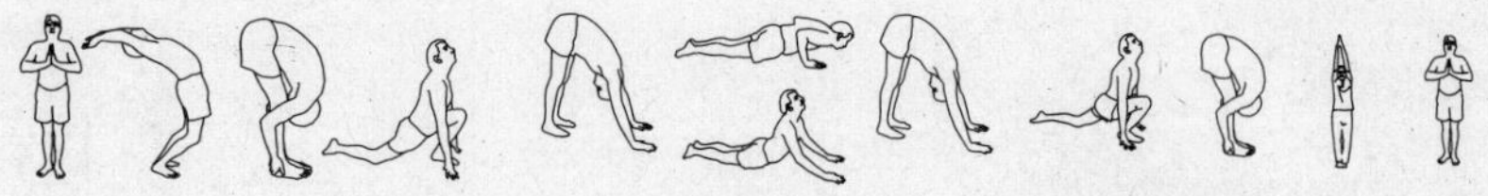

Pranayama

Surya Namaskar is a rhythmic expression of gratitude to the greatest deity of the universe. This is the biggest energy reservoir which refuels every time without asking for any paybacks. To the paradox of the usual give and take phenomenon, here it is only take and take on behalf of human beings when you perform this ritual to pay regards to the sun. You get in return a trio of physical, mental and spiritual harmonisation which is beautifully interlaced within the rhythmic patterns of this Surya Namaskar.

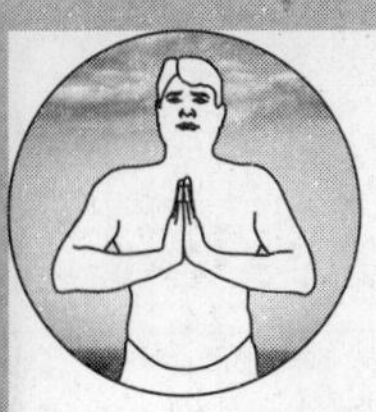

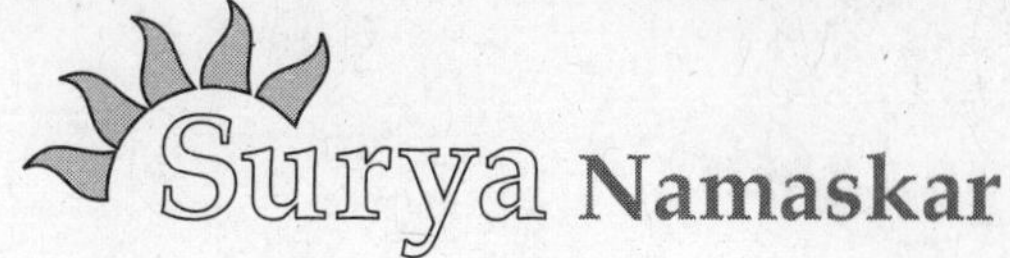

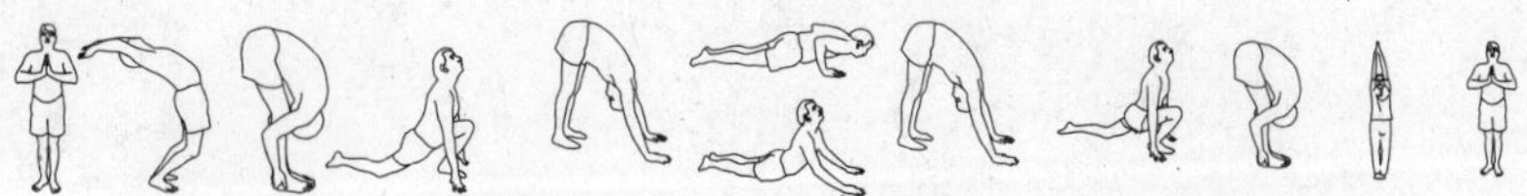

Surya Namaskar is actually performed at three different levels and is supposed to give similar impacts on

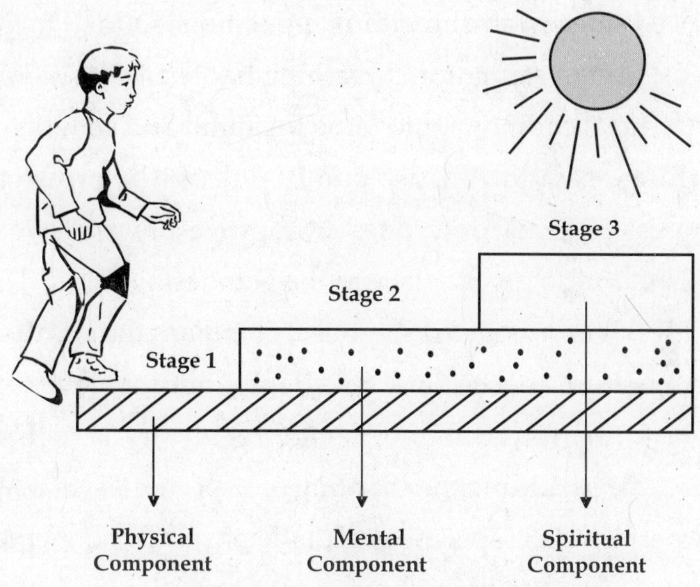

Stages of Surya Namaskar

the physical, mental and spiritual components of a person. The first level is the physical one which is a cyclical combination of different postures stressing every part of

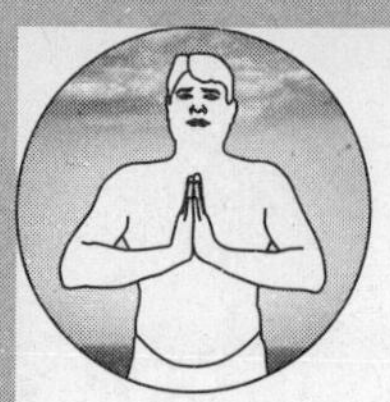

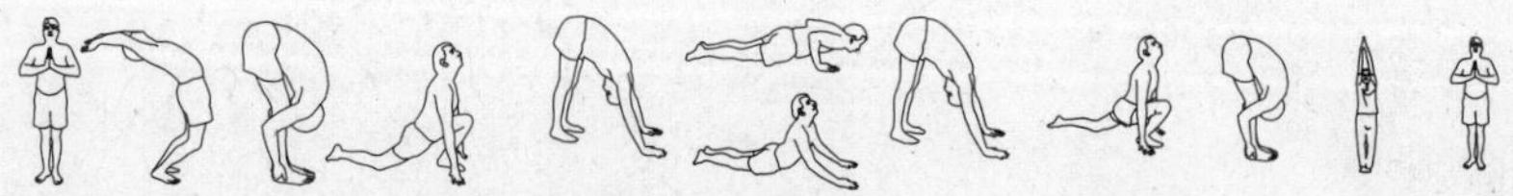

the body. This is the most commonly practised aspect of Surya Namaskar as it gives observable results in the form of physical fitness almost instantly. The second level is an advanced stage where breathing regulation is added to the physical part of salutation. Breathing has been considered a very crucial component to tame the mind and so when a breathing regulation is combined with physical harmonisation, not only does it improve physical well-being, but it also gives solace to the wandering mind. The third level is an advanced stage as it combines the spiritual component to the second level, i.e., adding spiritual activity to the physical and mental regulatory activities. This is done by adding the chanting of a specific *bija* mantra while performing a specific part of the physical and mental rhythm. This is the highest stage which unifies man with the universe even though transiently but whose impacts last forever.

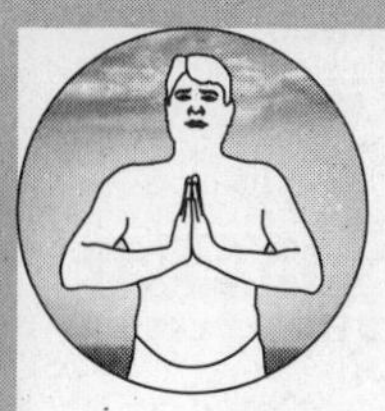

2. Before We Begin

This is stage one of Surya Namaskar which is earmarked by a series of rhythmic, cyclical and physical activities. These activities are supposed to stretch the whole body through a set of alternate opposite movements done within a short span of time. The benefits associated with this stage are not only related to the physical activities but also to the environment where these activities should be performed. The rising sun can dispel death. This is the endorsement given to the healing power of the sun at dawn by the *Atharvaveda* and *Ayurveda,* or the science of life. This endorsement has been beautifully exploited by the advocates of Surya Namaskar who have amalgamated the idea of physical exercise, the healing effects of the sun at dawn and the associated benefits of rising early in the morning.

Surya Namaskar is to be performed at dawn, in the open air, wearing clothes that absorb perspiration. There is no better way to imbibe the floating energy of nature to

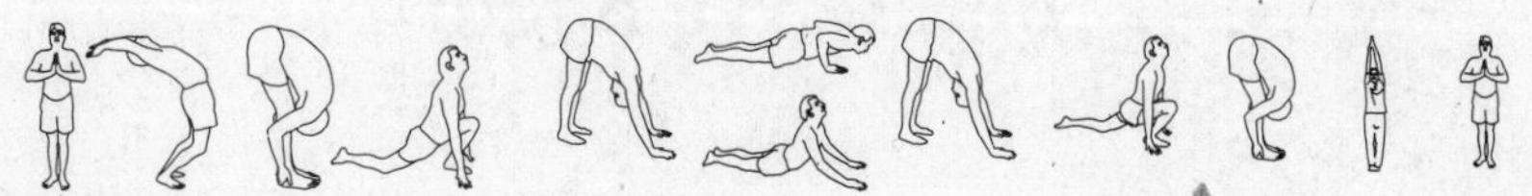

enrich one's own repository than Surya Namaskar. The biggest advantage associated with Surya Namaskar is that you get most of the benefits at the expense of time less than you take for brushing your teeth. Should this not be the kind of ritual which should be cherished?

It is nice to begin with the physical dimensions of Surya Namaskar as it gives instant results which are visible and, moreover, often these are the sole things which are desired by most people. Once you get accustomed to the beginner's stage, switching to more advanced stages becomes a matter of simple determination and will.

How to Begin

Before starting, it would be wise if we were to know of any situation where this is contraindicated and also the ideal situation where it can yield maximum benefits. Answers to some simple questions may give a better idea.

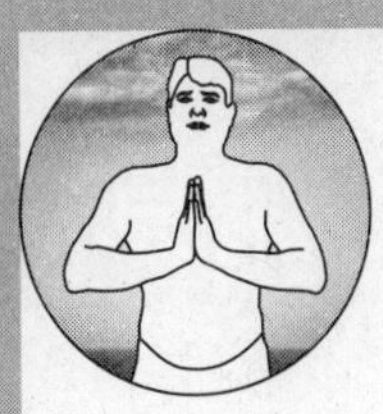

Surya Namaskar

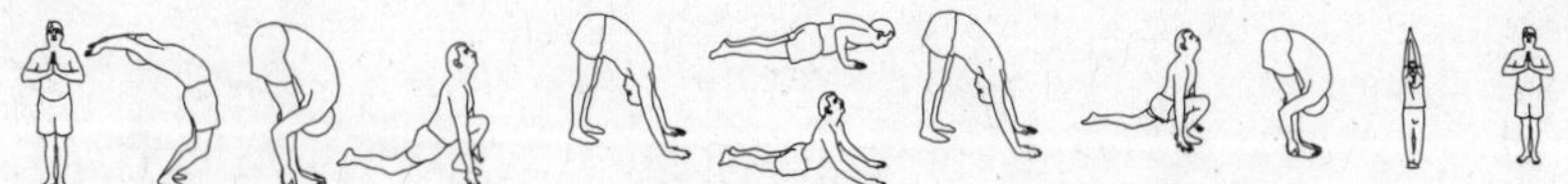

Who Can Do It

Every individual, who is active enough to perform the movements specified, can start Surya Namaskar. As the movements are intended to move the shoulder, elbow, knee, wrist, spine, hip and ankle joints, any limitation to these joints may limit the individual's capability to perform the rhythms correctly. Surya Namaskar does not have a sex bias or conditions applicable differentially to different people on the globe. It can be universally adopted by all people around the globe with a little modification, if required, depending on the individual conditions.

During Pregnancy

Surya Namaskar is permitted during the first trimester of pregnancy in its normal course. It is avoided during the advanced stages of pregnancy as the growing foetus and subsequent enlargement of the abdomen are constraints in performing the salutation correctly. In the

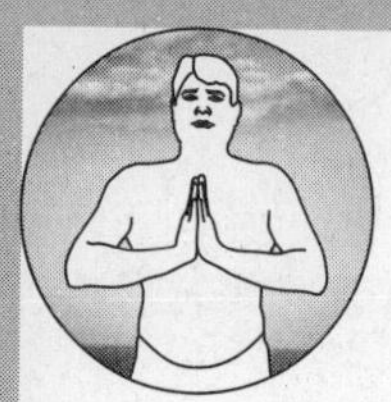

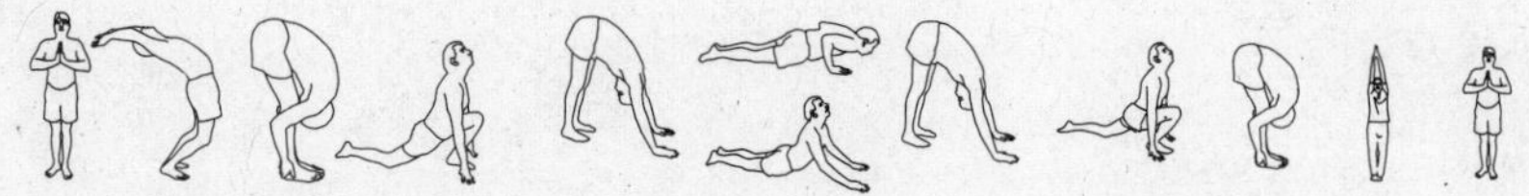

first trimester too, if it is a precious pregnancy, or if there is a history of miscarriage, it is better to avoid it or it should be done under the guidance of an experienced yoga therapist. In the normal course Surya Namaskar, may provide a calming and relaxing effect to the mother, especially those who are experiencing pregnancy for the first time. This can help in nullifying the anxiety and associated conditions like pregnancy-induced hypertension, and so can be helpful in the normal growth and subsequent delivery of the baby.

Post-Partum Period

Surya Namaskar may quickly be resumed once pregnancy is over. Surprisingly, this can help in uterus involution as a few specific movements in the salutation provide pressure massage to the uterus which can result in reduced congestion and reduction in uterus size. The relaxation associated with Surya Namaskar may be good to counteract post–partum anxieties and depression and may

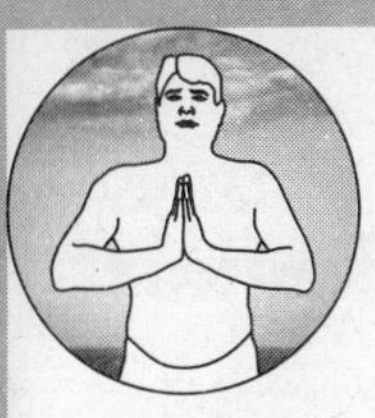

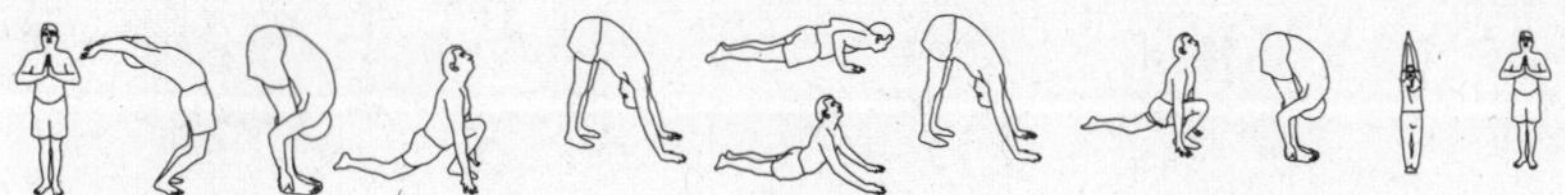

stimulate the neurochemical and immunological boosters which can help in safe and quick normalisation of the body's physiology. This can also have a positive impact upon the process of lactation. Care should be taken not to perform the activities to their full extent in the beginning as starting again after a long gap requires a period of acclimatisation to get accustomed to physical movements again. If it is an operative delivery, it is better to avoid the salutation for a period of six months so that the abdomen muscles can recover their strength. In the normal course, the period of puerparium (forty-five days after the delivery), moderate and supervised Surya Namaskar can be taken up and can help in reducing post-partum complications and help in improved physiology.

During Menstruation

There are no specific contraindications for stage one of Surya Namaskar during menstruation. The advanced stages are usually avoided on the basis of sanctity, in that

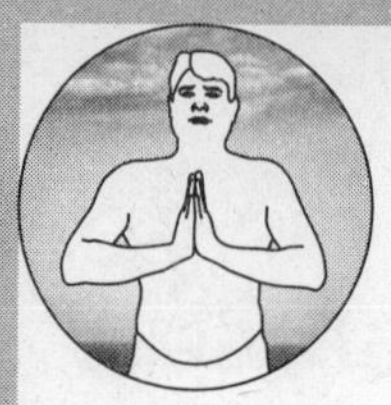

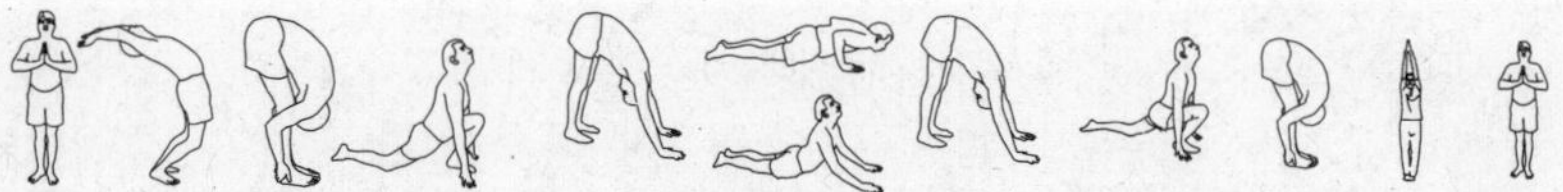

during menstruation, a woman does not feel clean enough to perform rituals attached to spirituality. Stage one salutation may also create a problem as in some of the movements, the lower abdomen is pressed, which may give rise to excessive bleeding to the vulnerable. It is best to avoid the salutation during this period and then to resume it quickly once it is over.

Which Age is the Best Age to Start?

Age is absolutely not a contraindication to start Surya Namaskar. It can be started at any age. The only caution to be observed is that the older you grow, the less resilient are your bones and joints. This simply limits the range of motion of the joints and makes bones vulnerable to stress fractures. This is more true for post-menopausal women where osteoporosis is a recognised condition. The golden rule is to start in moderation and then to increase the amplitude of exercise as much as the body permits. It is like bending a bamboo. The faster you try, greater are the

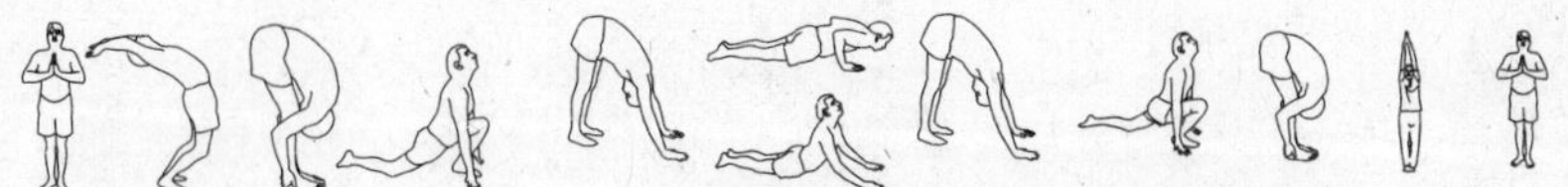

chances of breaking. On the contrary, if you bend it slowly, you can bend it to any shape you require. A moderately done Surya Namaskar may be good enough to reduce the loss of calcium from female bones and also help keeping the joints in shape. An early start at a younger age may also be associated with reduced risk of the conditions which are usually linked to people with a more sedentary lifestyle.

What is the Preferred Time to Practise?

As Surya Namaskar is essentially a prayer offered to the sun, it is imperative to perform it before the rise of the sun. Now which is the best time to do it between dawn and dusk? Dawn is considered the most sacred time. There are plenty of reasons for this, based upon scientific and religious theories but the most obvious is that this is the start of a fresh day and this could be the best time to imbibe natural energy from the reservoir of the universe.

Morning is the time for exacerbation of *kapha* (phlegm).

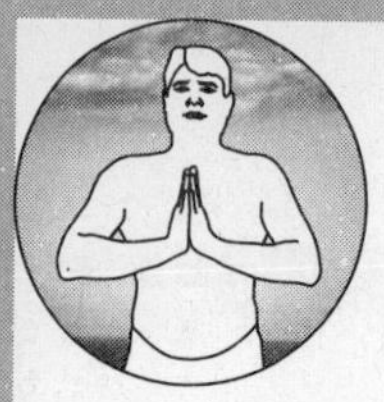

Surya Namaskar

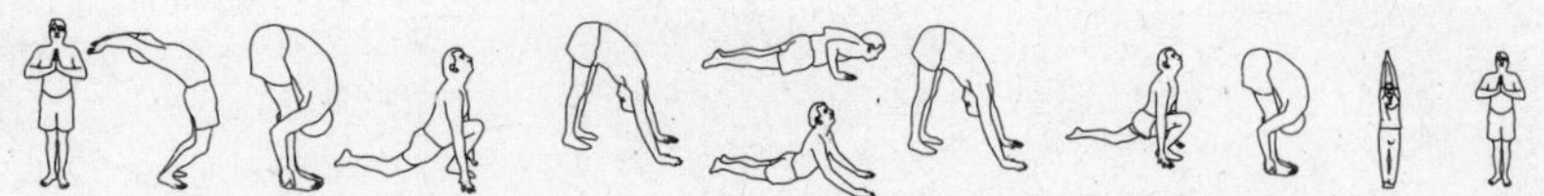

*A*ccording to the Ayurvedic Principles, night is the time when *kapha* accumulates and in the morning, it gets an opportunity to come out. This *kapha* in the present context is the resting secretions of the body especially to the tracheobronchial tree. During sleep as most of the reflexes are suppressed, these secretions don't get the opportunity to be expelled. Early morning cough reflexes are in accordance with this oriental wisdom which shows nature's effort to expel the accumulated secretions. Because of any reason if the cough reflex is suppressed (as in smokers and in the people living in a polluted environment) these secretions may go down along with all the contaminants they possess and start a pathogenesis. Surya Namaskar provides a wonderful opportunity to minimise these chances. Salutation done in front of the sun works as a two-pronged weapon to handle the situation. Heat provided by the sun added to the heat provided by physical movement (because of increased metabolic activity and thermogenesis) cumulatively dispels kapha.

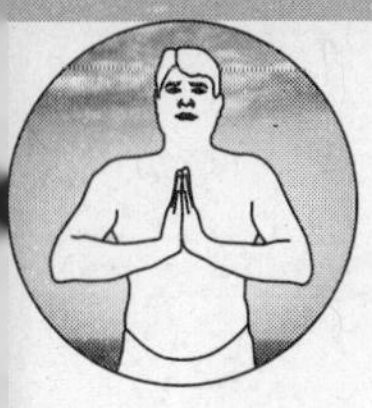

Surya Namaskar

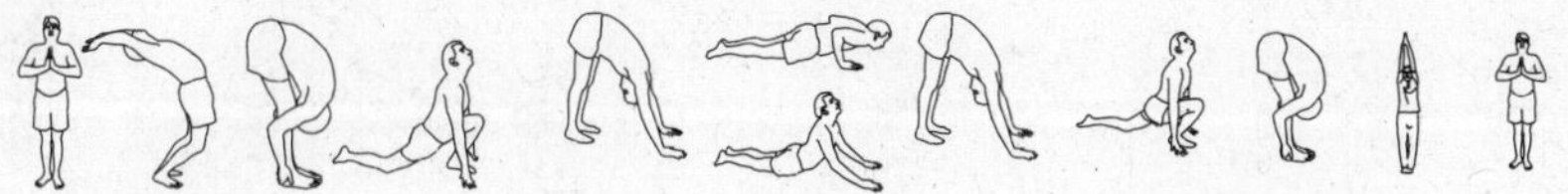

The *Vedas* are full of verses in praise of the rising sun. The *Atharvaveda* says that the rising sun has the capability to dispel death (*Atharvaveda 17.1.30*). It also says that the rays coming from the rising red-coloured sun are capable of curing heart diseases, jaundice and anemia and are able to provide a long, disease-free life (*Rigveda 1.50.11, Atharvaveda* 1.22.1-2). Sunrays have been said to be capable of destroying various disease-causing organisms including bacteria, viruses and moulds. This is why an area or an object exposed to sunrays is assumed to be free of disease-causing pathogens. It is a common practice in India to keep clothes and bed linen in direct sunlight for long hours if they are to be used after a long gap. The damp and exfoliated epithelial cells from the human body act as the most favourable environment for the growth of micropathogens responsible for various allergic responses to the human body including asthma and urticaria. Clothes used during a season and then kept for a long period of unuse act as the best habitat for these pathogens. Keeping

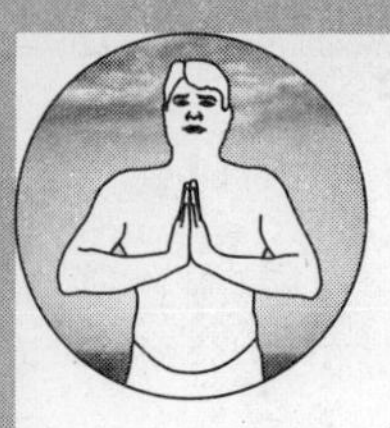

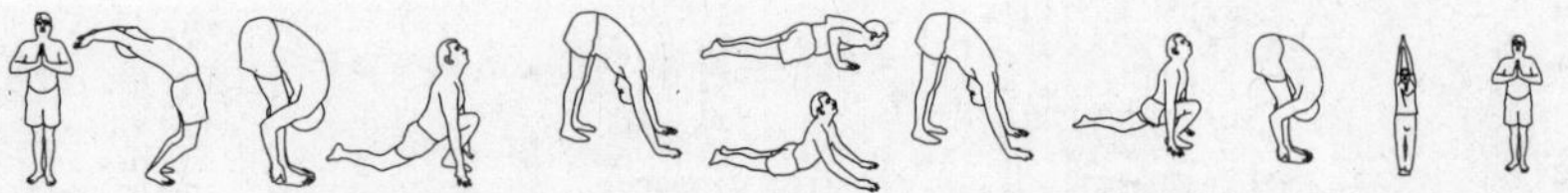

them in sunlight before they are reused is the best preventive practice observed in nature. The objects exposed to sunrays are considered as good as sterilised, at least empirically. Can we draw some benefits of Surya Namaskar by thinking along these lines?

Dawn and dusk are the only times when the sun can be visualised with unaided eyes. This is due to the mildness of the sunrays at these times. This mildness is mainly because of the relative long distance covered by sunrays to reach the earth's surface. The rays are coming horizontally above the earth's surface which increases their interaction with the suspended particles in the air and gives rise to the phenomenon of scattering. As a sunray is composed of seven independent wavelengths producing different coloured lights, those composed of shorter wavelengths are sorted out and defeated in the race to reach the earth. The longer wavelengths survive all the interactions and reach the earth. Orange and red are the longest

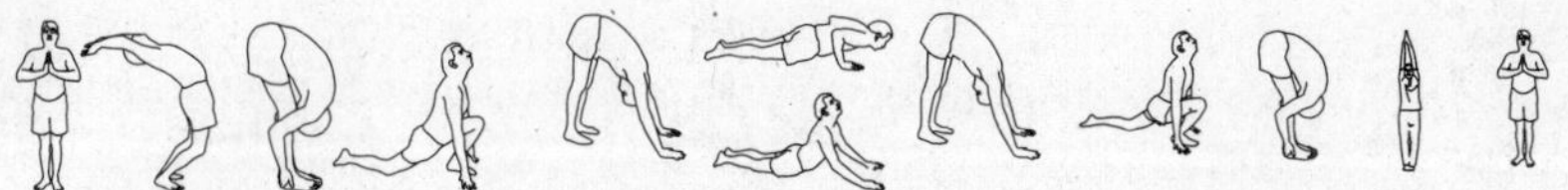

wavelengths in the visible solar spectrum and this is how we see the sun glowing red during dawn and dusk. There are many more reasons for performing the salutation in front of the rising sun. We will get a better idea as we proceed further.

What if We have Some Disease?

Unfortunately, health consciousness comes only when we fall sick. We only think of health preserving activities once we suffer the consequences of not following them. The biggest limiting factor for this is that we are not able to stretch the body as we should be able to. There are accompanying illnesses which act as restraints. It becomes difficult to decide what is good and what is not. Let us look at some diseases and see what is permissible and what is not.

Hypertension

A result of a hectic lifestyle, hypertension is common among most people who are over-stressed for any reason.

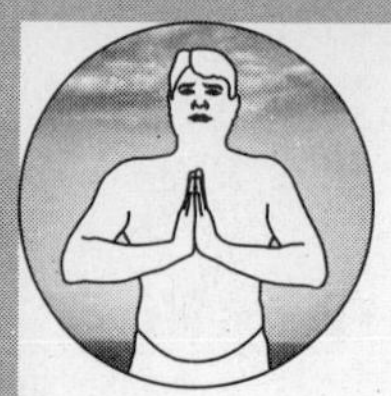

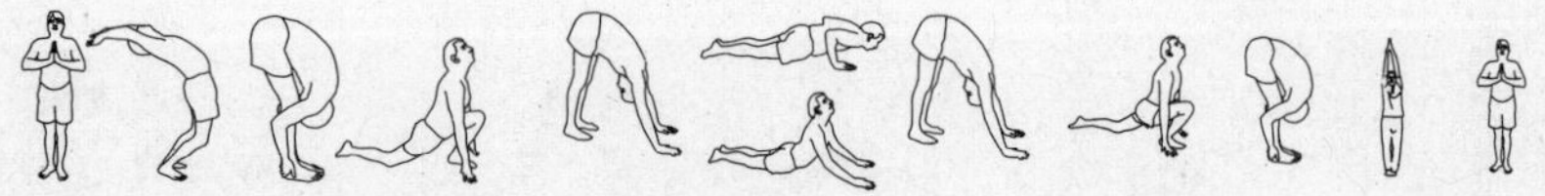

This can be overt where the symptoms show up or disguised and show up only when complications have set in. Surya Namaskar can be started with the medicines prescribed and it will be discovered later that gradually you require less of the medicine and can even live without them if the salutation is done perfectly. For the hypertensive, the paraphernalia of Surya Namaskar remains most important before the actual effect of the Surya Namaskar shows up. A calm, peaceful environment, early morning breeze and the tender warmth of the sun can make you completely relaxed even before you start the actual salutation. The only caution to be observed is that the movements should not be exhausting and it should be followed by a substantial period of rest or relaxation. At sunrise or even a little before that would be the ideal time for the hypertensive, as the further rising of the sun would be associated with increase in temperature which may not be beneficial to them.

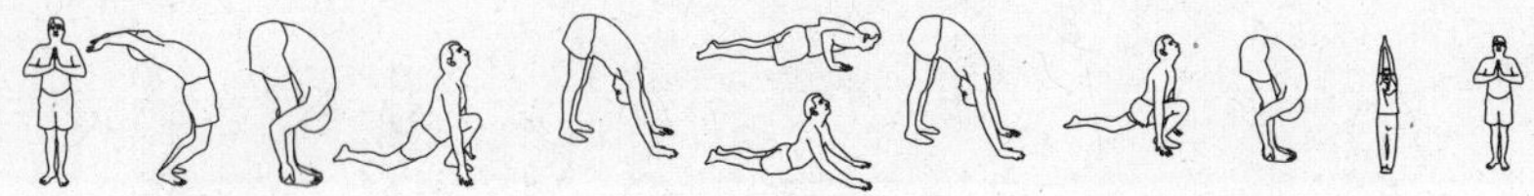

Diabetes

Maturity onset diabetes is again the disease of the common man now. The incidence is rising every year and it is taking the shape of an epidemic worldwide. A diabetic, if under control with his medication, should have no limitation in doing Surya Namaskar. However, the essential components of diabetes should always be kept in mind and the salutation should be performed accordingly. The place where this is being performed should be devoid of any stone or objects which can cause some trivial injury. Soft shoes can be worn and exposure to the sun should be limited to the early morning hours only as increasing heat may give rise to sunburn which may remain unnoticed because of hypersensitive skin. Some specific postures in the salutation which compress the abdomen, may stimulate the pancreas to secrete more insulin, which may reduce the requirement of medicine or insulin need for the control of diabetes. Moderate exercise of any kind is also

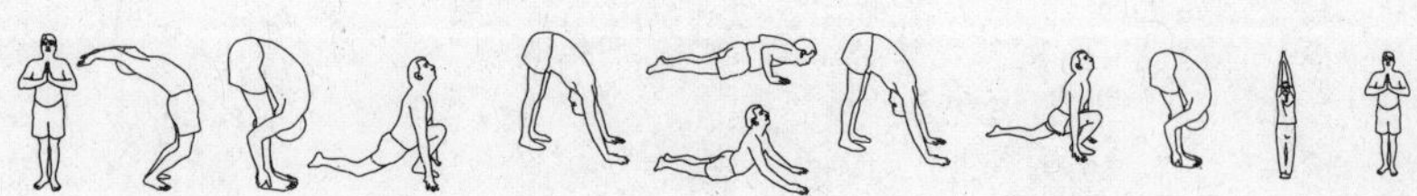

associated with increased insulin sensitivity and reduced insulin resistance, which also helps in better management of diabetes.

Depression

According to ancient wisdom, depression is caused by the dominance of *tama* (darkness) in the mind. Nothing other than the sun can be better to eliminate this *tama* from the mind. The physical activities, the warmth and increased metabolism associated with salutation, all lead to a better neurohormonal synchronisation in the mind which gives better stability to the mind. There are some parts of the brain which contain melanin pigments which have the capacity to absorb sunrays. They may also have some role to play in reducing depression. There are no contra-indications associated with depression while performing Surya Namaskar. The only vigilance to be observed is that it would be advisable if the ritual is performed by a group

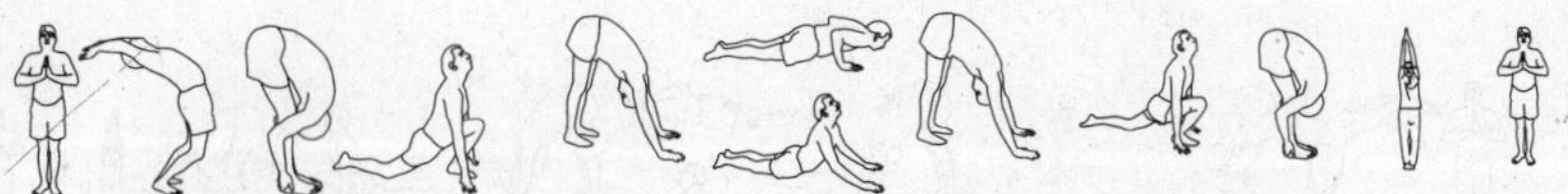

of people together. This would enable us to watch people performing the salutation and also help in deriving inspiration from them.

Vertigo

Vertigo may have a spectrum of causes. True vertigo which originates because of disturbances in the vestibulocochlear system of the internal ear, poses a problem in doing exercises where the head is lowered down. This may cause excess blood pooling in the ear and may lead to increased congestion which can cause some problem. Similarly, getting down on to the ground increases intra-abdominal pressure. As the ear is connected to the throat through the eustachian canal, any change in intra-abdominal pressure may affect the pressure status of the middle ear and may cause the tympanic membrane to protrude. In this condition, the lowering down activities are better avoided.

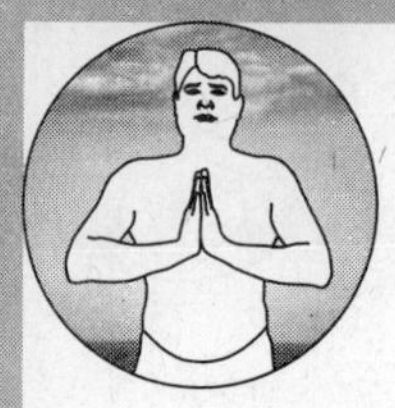

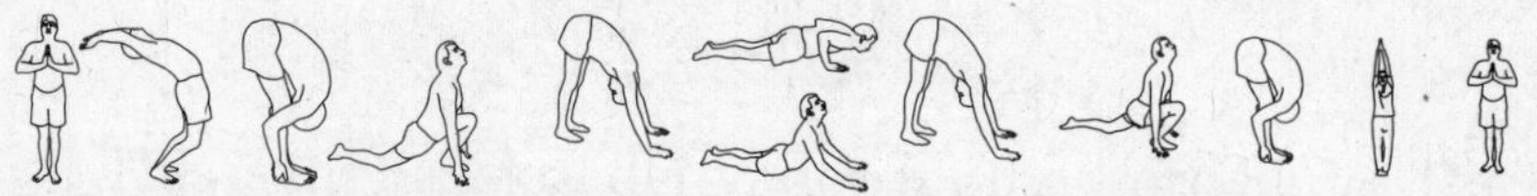

The Preferred Food

It is best to start Surya Namaskar on an empty stomach. As it involves activities which give rise to pressure on the intra-abdominal organs, a full stomach will be a hindrance to achieve the best effects of the internal massage. For diabetics or for other people who need to partake of something after waking up in the morning, a glass of lukewarm lemon water with some honey would suffice. Care should also be taken after the completion of the salutation not to consume a heavy meal immediately. At least a half-hour to one-hour interval is essential for the body metabolism to settle and food should only be eaten after that.

In the normal course too, the people who plan to get optimum benefit from Surya Namaskar are advised to have a diet which is minimal in calorie contents, fat and protein and preferably in its natural form unless it is contraindicated due to some reason.

3. The Ultraviolet Enigma

A lot has been said about ultraviolet radiation and its effects upon the body. As Surya Namaskar is to be performed in the sun and the emissions from the sun include light, heat and ultraviolet radiation, it would be wise to have an idea about these radiations and how they affect our body. The emissions from the sun have a broad range of wavelengths where the visible spectrum lies in the centre and ultraviolet radiations along with infrared radiations lie on the right and left sides respectively. The ultraviolet region of the spectrum covers the range of 100-400 nm and is sub-divided into 3 bands. These are :

UVA	315-400 nm
UVB	280-315 nm
UVC	100-280 nm

During the passage of sunlight through the atmosphere, all UVC and 90 per cent of the UVB radiation are absorbed by ozone, water vapour, oxygen and carbon

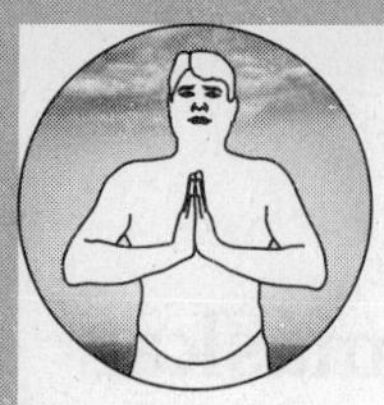

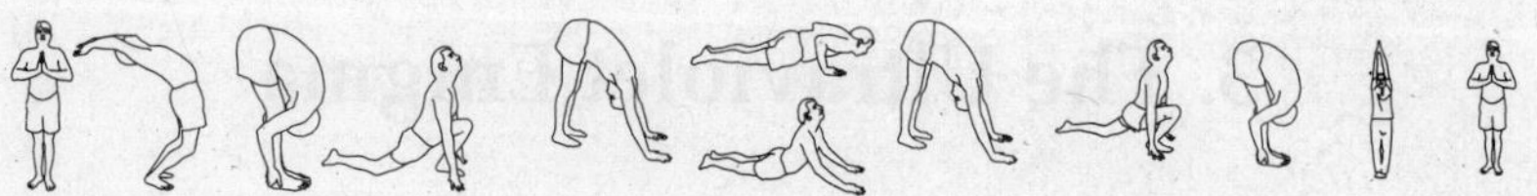

dioxide. UVA radiation is less affected by atmospheric variations and reaches the earth almost completely.

1. Ultra violet Climatology

The sun is responsible for the development and continued existence of life on earth. We are warmed by the sun's infrared rays and we can see with our eyes which respond to the visible part of the sun's terrestrial spectrum. More importantly, visible light is an essential component of photosynthesis, the process whereby plants, which are necessary for man's nutrition, derive their energy. However, the deleterious effects of sunlight on biological systems are due almost entirely to radiation within the ultraviolet spectrum of the sun's emission.

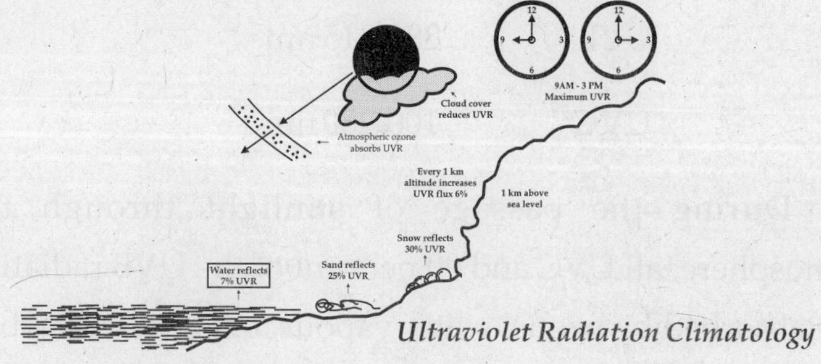

Ultraviolet Radiation Climatology

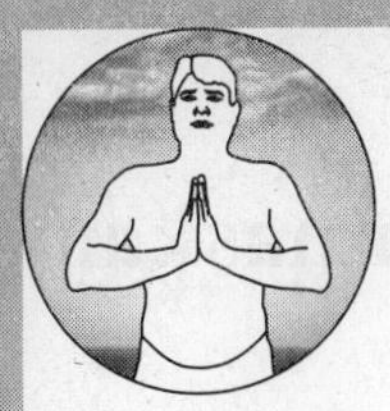

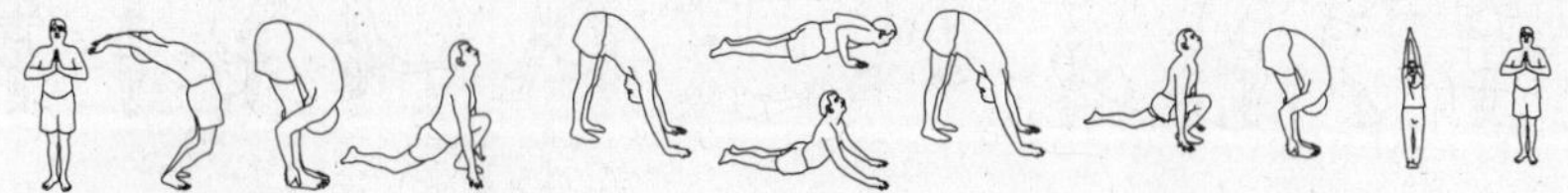

Atmospheric Ozone

The quality and quantity of ultraviolet radiation at the earth's surface depend on the energy output from the sun and the transmission properties of the atmosphere. From a biological viewpoint, UVB radiation is by far the most significant part of the terrestrial ultraviolet spectrum and the levels of radiation in this waveband reaching the surface of the earth are largely controlled by ozone, a gas which comprises approximately one molecule out of every two million in the atmosphere. Ozone (O_3) is created by the dissociation of oxygen (O_2) by short wavelength UVR (< 242 nm) in the stratosphere at altitudes between about 25 and 100 kms. Absorption of ultraviolet rays at wavelengths up to about 320 nm converts the O_3 back to O_2 and O. Dissociation of O_3 is the mechanism responsible for preventing radiation at wavelengths less than about 290 nm from reaching the earth's surface. It is increasingly realised that chlorofluorocarbons (CFCs) and other gases released by human activities alter the natural balance of

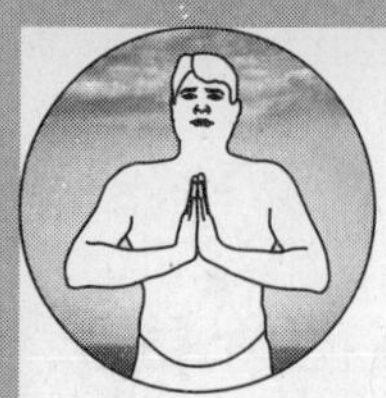

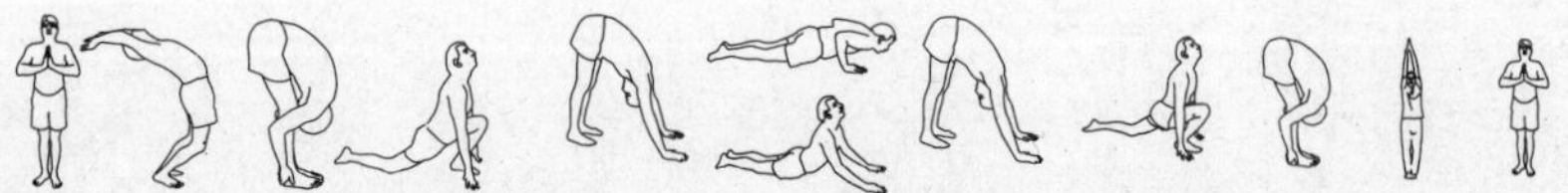

creative and destructive processes and lead to depletion of the stratospheric ozone layer. Substantial reductions of up to 50 per cent in the ozone column observed in the austral spring over Antarctica first reported in 1985 is still continuing. Coupled with this, there has been a statistically significant downward trend in wintertime total ozone over the northern hemisphere of about 2-3 per cent per decade for the past 30 years, although summertime ozone levels have remained approximately constant.

Factors Affecting Terrestrial Ultraviolet Rays

The spectral irradiance of ultraviolet rays at the earth's surface is modified by temporal, geographical and meteorological factors. In the ultraviolet region, spectral irradiance falls by a factor of only two or three as the wavelength decreases from 400 to 320 nm at solar altitudes higher than 20 degrees and then drops rapidly by three orders of magnitude or more from 320 to 290 nm as absorption by stratospheric ozone becomes important.

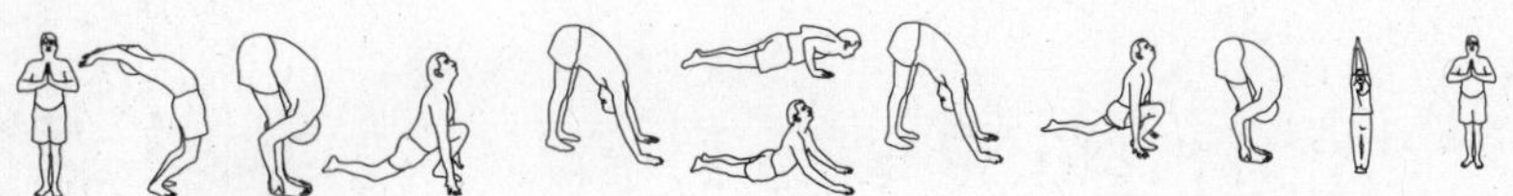

Time of Day

About 20-30 per cent of the total ultraviolet rays are received daily one hour before and after midday in summer, and 75 per cent between 9 a.m. and 3 p.m.

Season

In temperate regions, the biologically damaging ultraviolet rays reaching the earth's surface show strong seasonal dependence. However, seasonal variation is much less near the equator.

Geographical Latitude

Annual ultraviolet rays flux decreases with increasing distance from the equator.

Clouds

Clouds reduce solar irradiance at the earth's surface although changes in the ultraviolet region are not as great

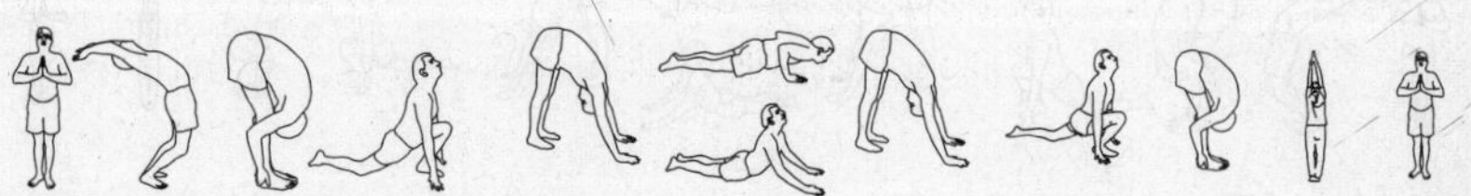

as those of total intensity, since water in clouds attenuates solar infrared much more than ultraviolet rays. The risk of overexposure may be increased under these conditions because the warning sensation of heat is diminished.

Light clouds scattered over a blue sky make little difference to ultraviolet rays intensity unless directly covering the sun, while complete light cloud cover reduces terrestrial ultraviolet rays to about one–half of that from a clear sky. Even with heavy cloud cover, the scattered ultraviolet component of sunlight (often called skylight) is seldom less than 10 per cent of that under a clear sky. However, very heavy storm clouds can virtually eliminate terrestrial ultraviolet rays even in summer time.

Surface Reflection

Reflection of ultraviolet rays from ground surfaces, including the sea, is normally low (less than 7 per cent). However, gypsum sand reflects about 25 per cent of incident UVB and fresh snow about 30 per cent.

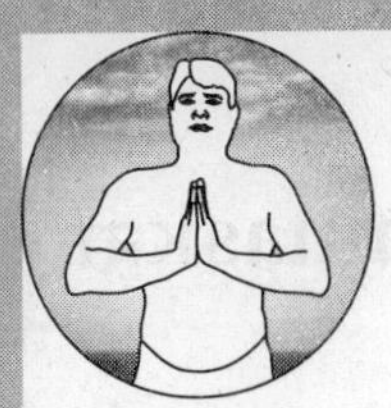

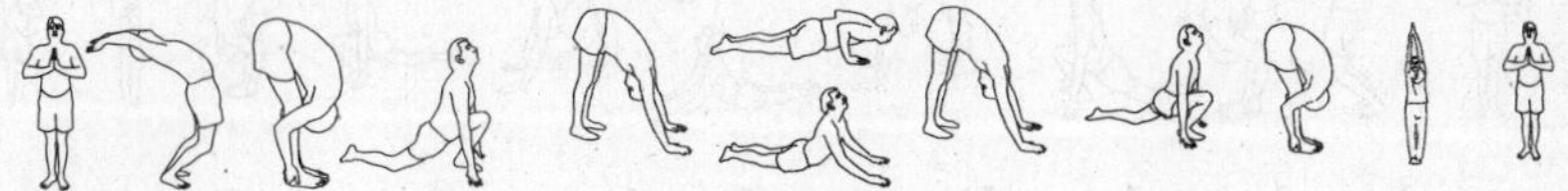

Altitude

In general, each kilometre increase in altitude increases the ultraviolet flux by about 6 per cent. Conversely, places on the earth's surface below sea level are relatively poorer in UVB content than sites at sea level. This is strikingly apparent around the Dead Sea in Israel, 400 nm below sea level.

2. Effects of Solar Ultraviolet Rays on Humans

The observable biological effects in man due to exposure from solar ultraviolet rays are limited to the skin and to the eyes because of the low penetrating properties of ultraviolet rays in human tissues. The penetration into skin is less than one mm and ultraviolet rays are absorbed by ocular tissues (mainly the cornea and the lens) before it reaches the retina.

Effects of Solar Ultraviolet Rays on Normal Skin

The normal responses of the skin to ultraviolet rays

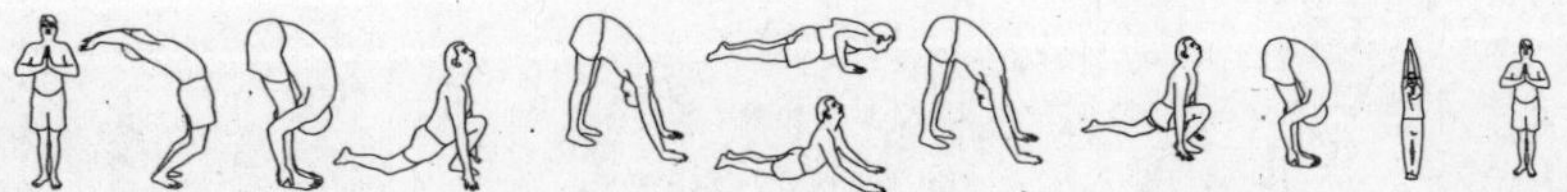

can be classed under two headings: acute effects and chronic effects. An acute effect is one of rapid onset and generally of short duration, as opposed to a chronic effect

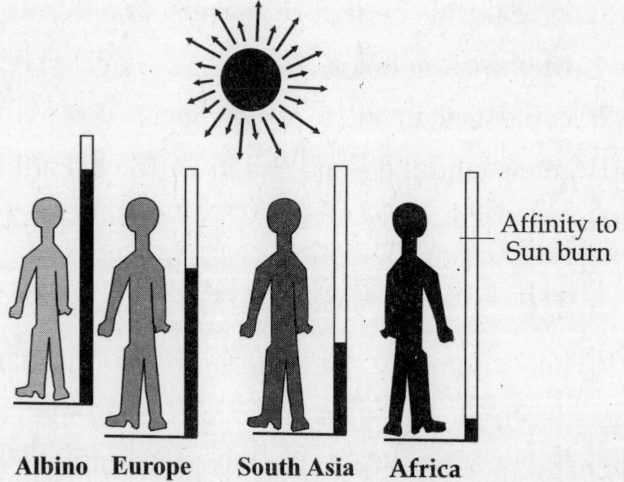

Affinity to Develop Sunburn in Different Skin Types

which is often of gradual onset and of long duration. These effects should be distinguished from acute and chronic exposure conditions which refer to the length of exposure to the ultraviolet rays. The acute reactions considered will be sunburn, tanning and vitamin D production. Photo-

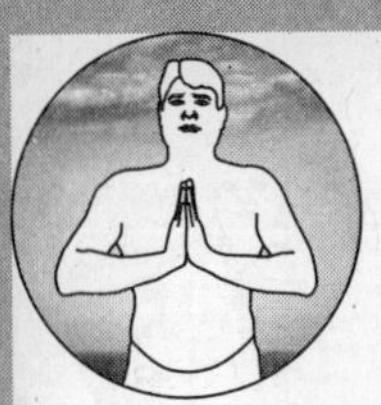

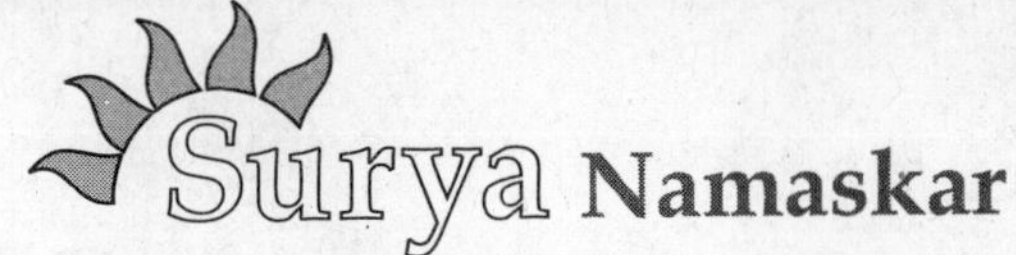

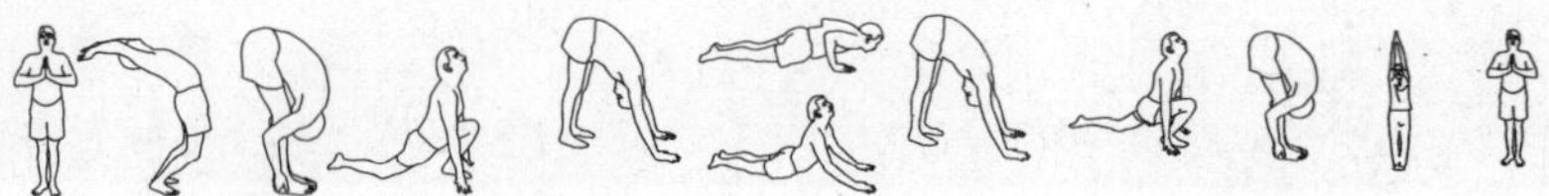

ageing and skin cancer will be discussed as those chronic reactions produced by prolonged or repeated ultraviolet rays exposure.

Sunburn

Sunburn, or erythema, is an acute injury following excessive exposure to solar ultraviolet rays. The redness of the skin which results is due to an increased blood content of the skin by dilatation of the superficial blood vessels in the dermis, mainly the sub-papillary venuels.

Time Course of Sunburn

Half an hour of midday summer sunshine in the UK on the unacclimatised skin of Caucasian subjects is normally sufficient to result in a mild reddening of the skin. Following this degree of exposure, erythema may not appear for about four hours, although measurements using an instrument more sensitive than the eye at detecting erythema showed that vasodilatation begins to

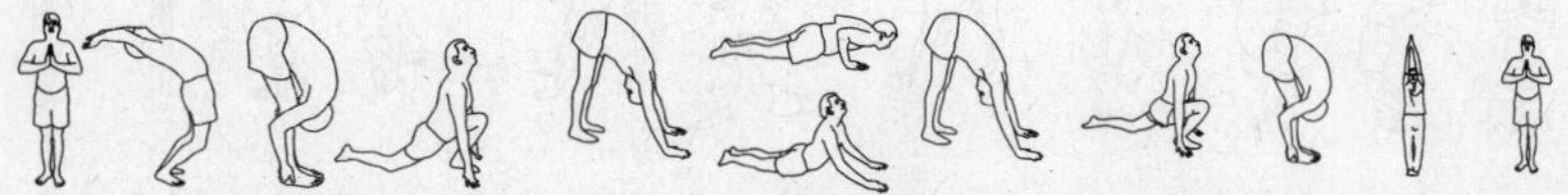

occur much sooner. The erythema reaches a maximum around eight to twelve hours after exposure and fades within one to two days. Exposing the skin for increasing periods to strong summer sunshine progressively shortens the time before the appearance of erythema, lengthens its persistence and increases its intensity. High doses may result in edema, pain, blistering, and after a few days, peeling.

Factors Influencing the Development of Sunburn

Skin colour is an important factor in determining the ease with which the skin will get sunburnt. Whereas fair-skinned people require only about fifteen to thirty minutes of midday summer sunshine to induce an erythemal reaction, people with moderately pigmented skin may require an exposure of one to two hours, while those with darkly pigmented skin (i.e. Blacks) will not normally get sunburnt. Other phenotype characteristics that may influence the susceptibility to sunburn are hair colour, eye colour and freckles. Based on a personal history of

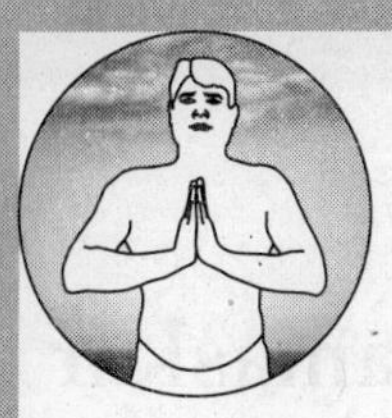

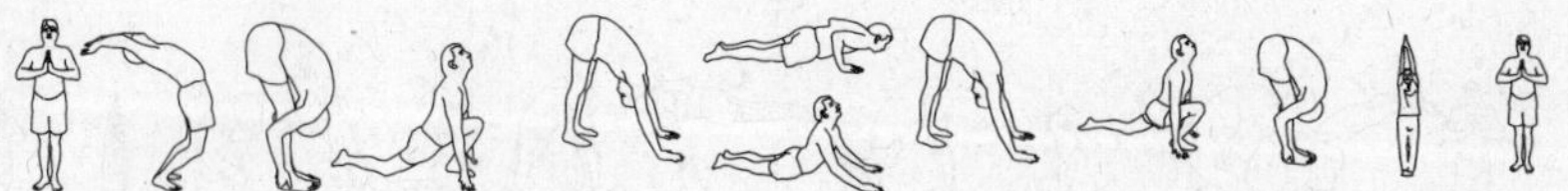

response to forty-five to sixty minutes of exposure to midday summer sun in early June, individuals can be grouped into six sun-reactive skin types.

There are anatomical differences in erythemal sensitivity. The face, neck and trunk are two to four times more sensitive than the limbs. These anatomical differences are compounded by the variations in solar exposure on different parts of the body. Vertical surfaces of an upright person receive about one half of the ambient ultraviolet rays, whereas horizontal surfaces, such as the epaulet region of the shoulder, receive up to 75 per cent.

There is no difference in sunburn susceptibility between sexes, although erythemal sensitivity may change with age, in that young children and elderly people are said to be more sensitive.

Sunburn and Epidermal Thickening

In addition to erythema and tanning, thickening (hyperplasia) of the epidermis is a significant component

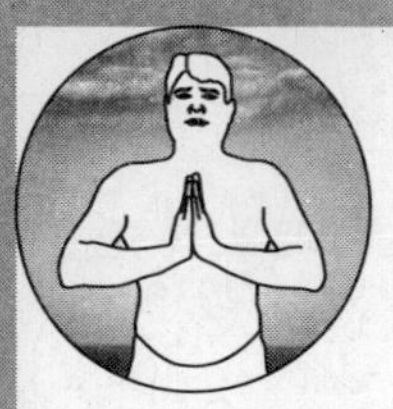

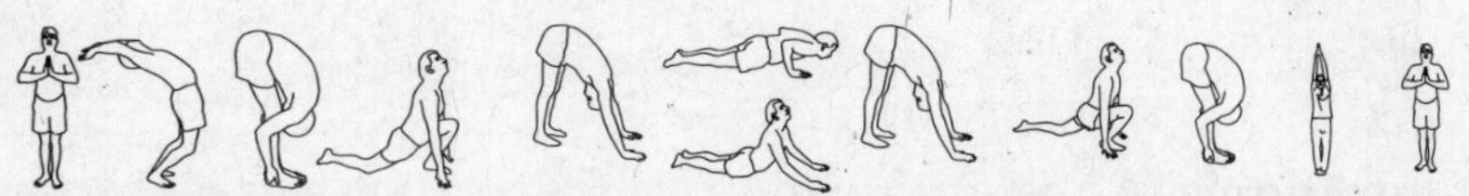

of a mild sunburn reaction. A single moderate exposure to UVB can result in up to a three-fold thickening of the stratum corneum, the outermost layer of the skin within one to three weeks, and multiple exposures every one to two days for up to seven weeks will thicken the stratum corneum by about three- to five-fold. Skin thickness returns to normal in about one to two months after ceasing irradiation.

Thickening of the skin, especially of the stratum corneum, after sun exposure, can lead to a significant increase in protection against ultraviolet rays by a factor of five or even higher. In Caucasians, skin thickening is probably more important than tanning in providing endogenous photo protection, although in darkly pigmented races, it is likely that skin pigmentation is the most important means of protection against solar ultraviolet rays.

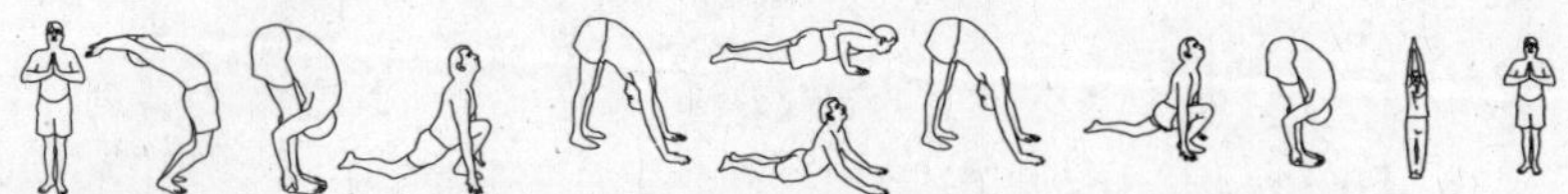

Tanning

A socially desirable consequence of exposure to unfiltered sunlight is the increased pigmentation of the skin known as tanning. Melanin pigmentation of skin is of two types: constitutive—the colour of the skin seen in different races and determined by genetic factors only; and facultative—the reversible increase in tanning in response to solar ultraviolet rays (and other external stimuli).

Immediate Pigment Darkening (IPD)

This is a transient darkening of exposed skin which can be induced by UVA and visible radiation. In general, the greater the constitutive tan, the greater is the ability to exhibit IPD. Immediate tanning can become evident within five to ten minutes of exposure to summer sun and normally fades within one to two hours.

Delayed Tanning

The more familiar delayed tanning becomes

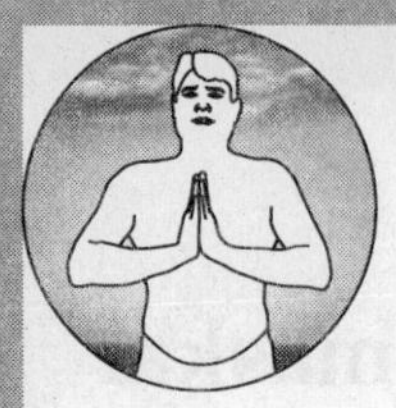

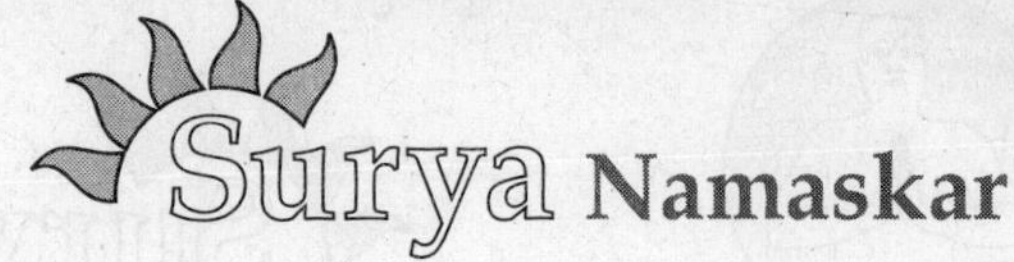

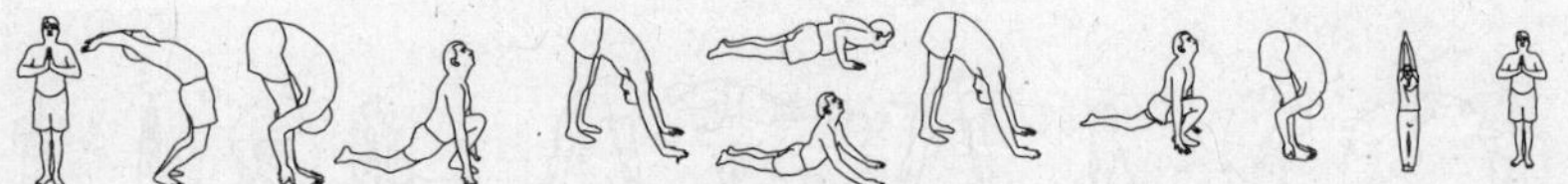

noticeable about one to two days after exposure to the sun, gradually increases for several days and may persist for weeks or months.

Following solar exposure to ultraviolet rays there is an increase in the number of functioning melanocytes and the activity of the enzyme tyrosinase is enhanced. This leads to the formation of new melanin and hence an increase in the number of melanin granules throughout the epidermis.

Although a tanned skin does confer a degree of photo protection, such protection seems to be no more than moderate, a factor of only two to three being achieved by a deep UVA-induced tan in the absence of skin thickening. Melanin is not an effective sunscreen for Caucasian skin and it has been suggested that, contrary to popular belief, melanin is not an evolutionary adaptation to protect humans from the damaging effects of sunlight. Instead, it is postulated that hominids developed melanin as a camouflage and as a device to keep their bodies warm in a forest environment.

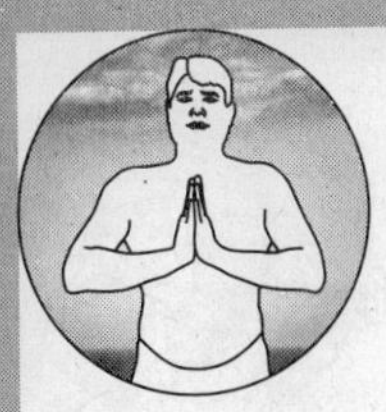

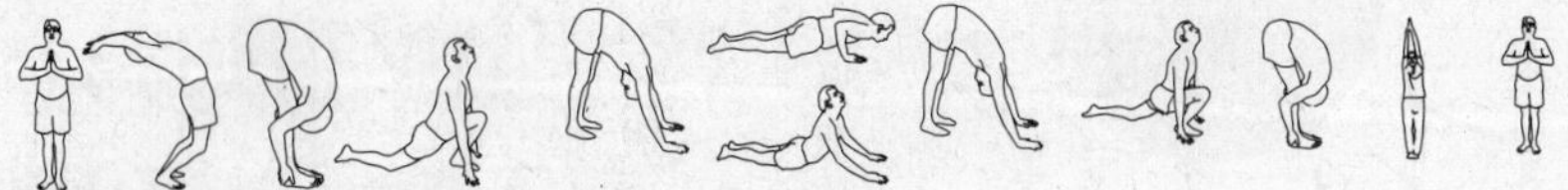

Production of Vitamin D3

The only thoroughly established beneficial effect of solar ultraviolet radiation on the skin is the synthesis of vitamin D3. Solar radiation in the UVB waveband photo chemically converts 7-dehydrocholesterol in the epidermis to previtamin D3. This previtamin immediately isomerises to vitamin D3 in a reaction controlled by skin temperature, which takes two to three days to reach completion. Previtamin D3 is photo labile and excessive exposure to sunlight causes its photolysis to the biologically inert photoproducts, lumisterol and tachysterol. In fact, production of previtamin D3 is limited to no more than 5-15 per cent of the total 7-dehydrocholesterol content in the skin, no matter how long a person is exposed to sunlight. Once vitamin D3 is made in the skin, it enters the blood for transport to the liver to be metabolised to 25-hydroxyvitamin D. If vitamin D3 does not enter the circulation before sun exposure the following day, it can be

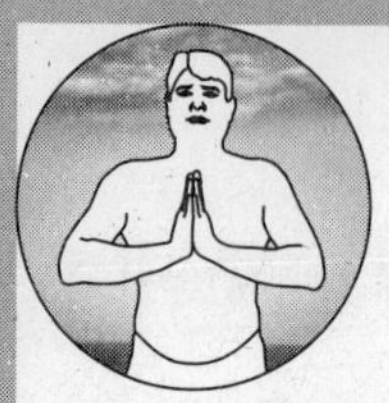

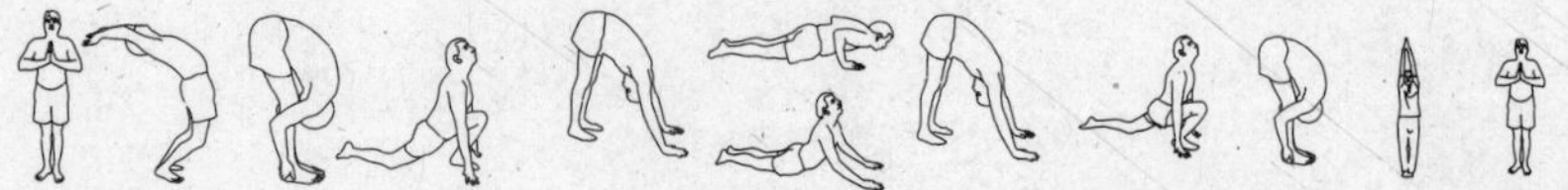

rapidly degraded in the skin by sunlight to biologically inert products. Thus sunlight, through its photochemical activity, is able to regulate the production of both previtamin D3 and vitamin D3 in the skin.

Only short exposures to sunlight are required to synthesise vitamin D3 in the skin; from spring until autumn an exposure of fifteen minutes to the hands, arms and face between 9 a.m. and 4 p.m. is adequate to provide our vitamin D3 requirements. Increased melanin pigmentation in the skin can limit the production of vitamin D3 as can increasing age. It is not surprising, therefore, that the seasonal variation of solar UVB, and hence plasma 25-hydroxyvitamin D3 levels can lead to calcium imbalance in the elderly.

Photo-ageing

The clinical signs of a photo-aged skin are dryness, deep wrinkles, accentuated skin furrows, sagging, loss of elasticity, mottled pigmentation and telangiectasia. These

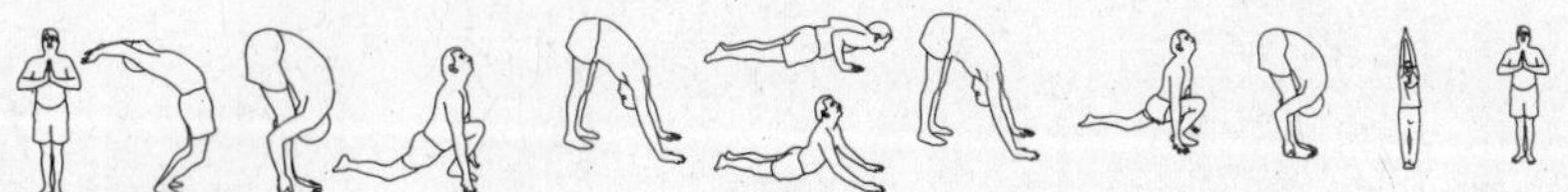

characteristics reflect profound structural changes in the dermis. It has been speculated that perhaps as much as 80 per cent of solar ultraviolet-induced photo-ageing occurs within the first 20 years of life, with the exception of those whose occupations or lifestyles result in extensive exposure as adults.

Prevention/Reversal of Photo-ageing

The application of topical sun screens has been shown to inhibit photo-ageing for those people chronically exposed to simulated solar radiation. It has been argued that the incorporation of sunscreens into products used for daily cosmetic care could markedly delay the onset of photo-ageing, as well as reduce the risk of skin cancer. Now as the importance of UVA in photo-ageing is recognised, it will be important to use sunscreens that incorporate ingredients which provide photo protection against both UVB and UVA. Photo-aged skin has the capacity to repair ultraviolet rays-induced connective tissue damage and it

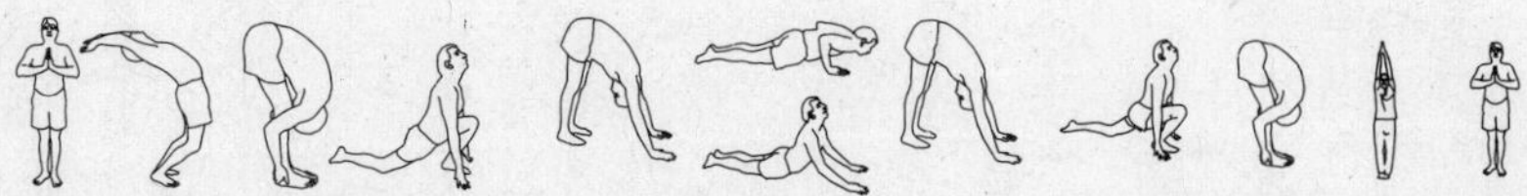

has been shown that topical retinoic acid can enhance this process and improve photo-aged skin.

Non-melanoma Skin Cancer

Skin cancer is the most common human cancer and there is little dispute that chronic exposure to solar ultraviolet radiation is the most important cause of non-melanoma skin cancers (NMSC). The two common types of NMSC are basal cell carcinoma (BCC) and squamous cell carcinoma (SCC). BCC accounts for about 80 per cent of all NMSC. The evidence for the carcinogenic effects of solar ultraviolet rays is discussed below.

Anatomical Distribution

About 90 per cent of all BCC and more than half of all SCC occur on the head and neck.

Racial Differences

Caucasians are much more likely to develop NMSC than races with more marked pigmentation. Furthermore,

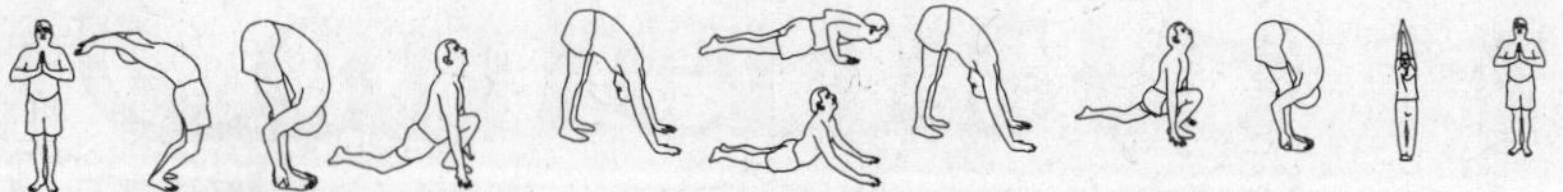

when skin cancer does occur in pigmented races, it is not found predominantly on light exposed areas.

Phenotype

Genetic factors associated with a tendency to develop skin cancer are light eyes, fair complexion, light hair colour, tendency to sunburn and poor ability to tan.

Geographical Distribution

Surveys of the incidence of skin cancer carried out in various countries yield ample evidence that a geographical latitude gradient exists. Very roughly, the incidence doubles for every 10 degree decrease in latitude, provided that the population is genetically equally susceptible. NMSC is essentially a disease of the elderly.

Occupation

Studies have shown that people who work outdoors are more likely to develop skin cancer than indoor workers.

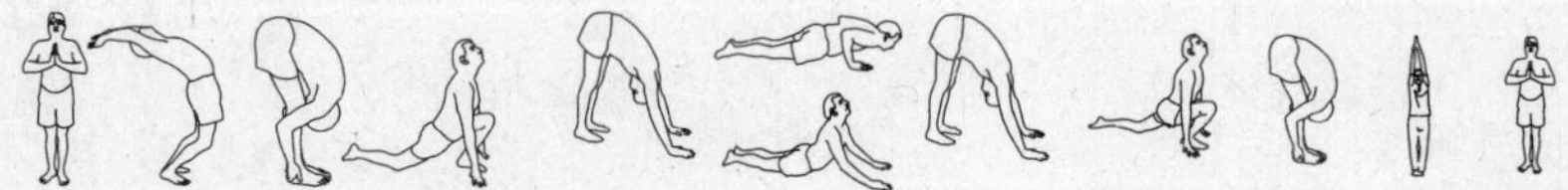

Malignant Melanoma

Malignant melanoma is a tumour derived from the pigment cells (melanocytes) of the skin. Unlike NMSC, melanomas have a marked tendency to metastasise. In the USA, melanoma incidence has almost doubled in the past decade and in Sweden, there was a five-fold increase in incidence between 1958 and 1984. Changing patterns of sun exposure are believed to be an important factor in the continuing rise in incidence. Some of the features of melanoma incidence are summarised below.

Geographical Distribution

In general, there is an inverse relationship between melanoma incidence and latitude of residence.

Racial Differences

Melanoma is much more common in Caucasians than in heavily pigmented races despite the fact that the latter tend to live in sunnier climates. An obvious explanation for

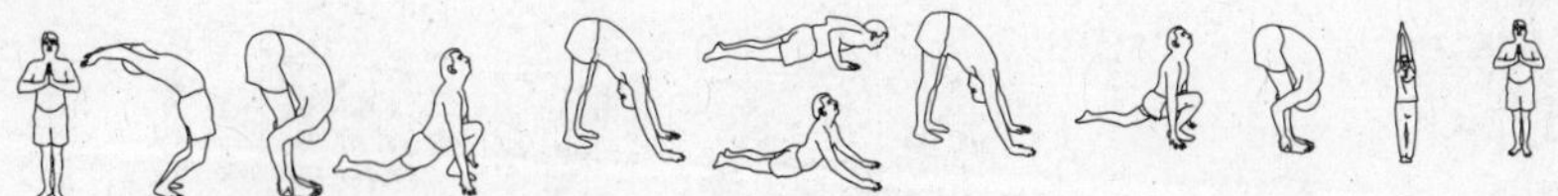

this is that the greater degree of epidermal melanin found in the skin of darker races protects melanocytes in the basal layer of the epidermis from the harmful effects of solar ultraviolet rays.

Phenotype

The single most important risk factor for developing melanoma is the total number of naive (moles) larger than 2 mm diameter. Blue eyes, blond or red hair, light complexion and tendency to sunburn are other risk factors.

Anatomical Distribution

Unlike NMSC, which predominates on sites of highest insolation (head, neck and hands), melanoma occurs much more frequently on the trunk and legs.

Occupation and Social Status

Melanoma is more common in professional and technical indoor workers than in those who work

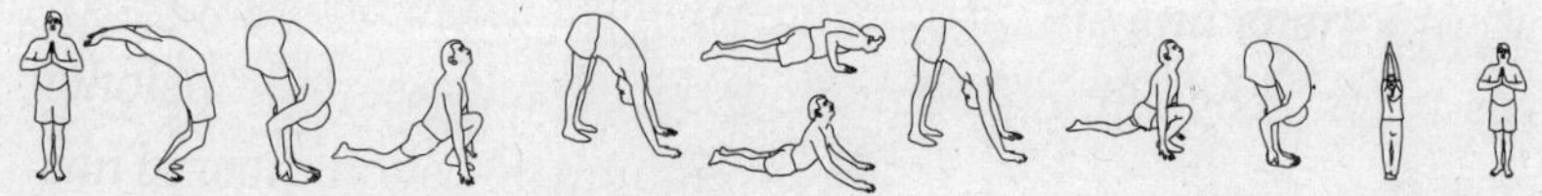

outdoors, such as farmers. Unlike all other cancers, melanoma is more likely to occur to those belonging to a higher socio-economic status.

Migration and Critical Period Studies

People born in Europe and who migrate to sunnier countries such as Israel, Australia or New Zealand after childhood have a higher risk of developing melanoma compared to a quarter of people of European descent born in those countries. However, arrival during childhood results in a comparable risk. This observation suggests that sun exposure during childhood plays a crucial role in the etiology of melanoma.

Intermittent Exposure Hypothesis

Although the evidence from epidemiological studies indicates an association between melanoma and sunlight exposure, it does not appear that cumulative sun exposure

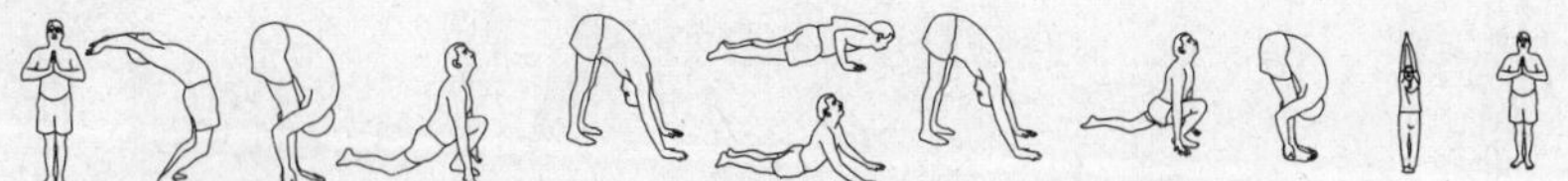

explains the relationship, as it does for NMSC. Instead, an intermittent exposure hypothesis proposes that infrequent intense exposure of unacclimatised skin to sunlight is related to increasing melanoma incidence and is more important than chronic sun exposure. This hypothesis is supported by the observation that most studies have shown that an increased risk of melanoma is associated with a past history of severe sunburn in childhood and adolescence.

Effects of Solar Ultraviolet Rays on the Eye

Effects on the Cornea

The association between UVB exposure and photokeratitis, or snow blindness, has been established for some time. Ambient levels of solar ultraviolet rays are such that this acute phototoxic corneal disorder is largely confined to snowfields and deserts. It has been estimated that approximately two hours of exposure outdoors

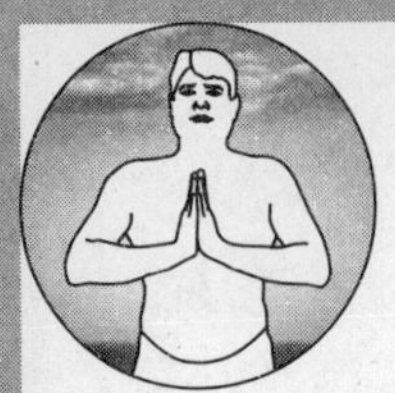

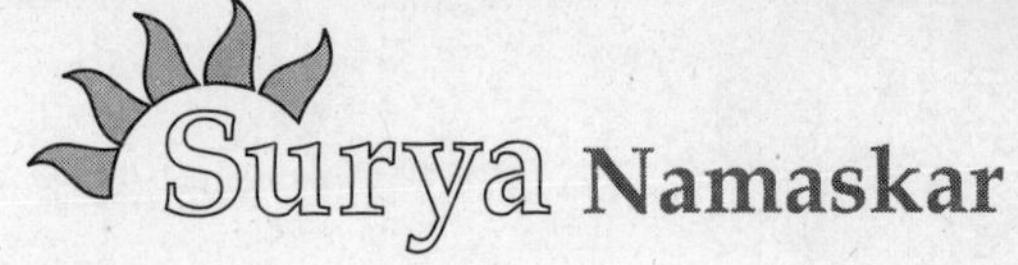

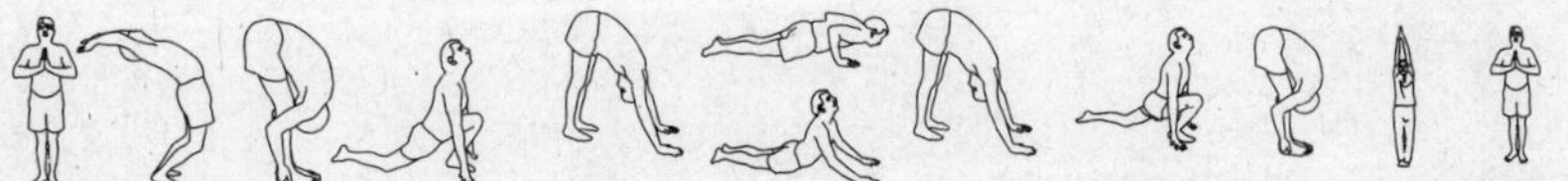

around noon on snow-covered terrain is sufficient to induce photokeratitis, and that of an exposure of six to eight hours in sandy terrain.

It has been shown recently that outdoor workers with high solar exposure have an approximate three-fold risk of developing pterygium (a fleshy growth on a normally clear cornea) and a six-fold risk of having climatic droplet keratopathy (a deposition of altered proteins on the superficial cornea leading to opacification).

Effects on the Lens

Studies have confirmed that the development of certain types of cataract (opacity of the lens) is associated with ocular UVB exposure.

Effects on the Retina

No association of senile macular degeneration has been found with solar UVB exposure.

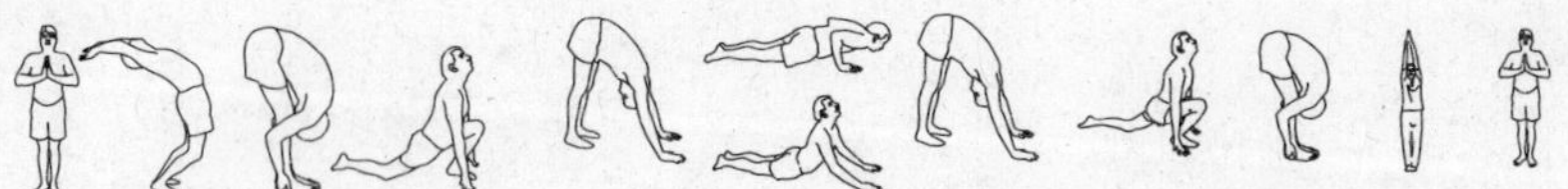

Implications of Ultraviolet Rays upon Surya Namaskar

As Surya Namaskar is essentially performed in the sun, the possible implications of ultraviolet rays while practising it, raises a point of concern in the informed mind. The things which are to be considered are:

1. Surya Namaskar should essentially be performed at dawn as at this time, the ultraviolet radiation falling on earth is minimal.

2. If it is performed when the sun is at a height, it should be done in the shade and not in direct sunlight. This will prevent undue exposure from the deleterious effects of the ultraviolet rays.

3. Rise in altitude results in an increase in intensity of ultraviolet radiation. So, for people living at higher altitudes, direct exposure to the midday sun should be avoided.

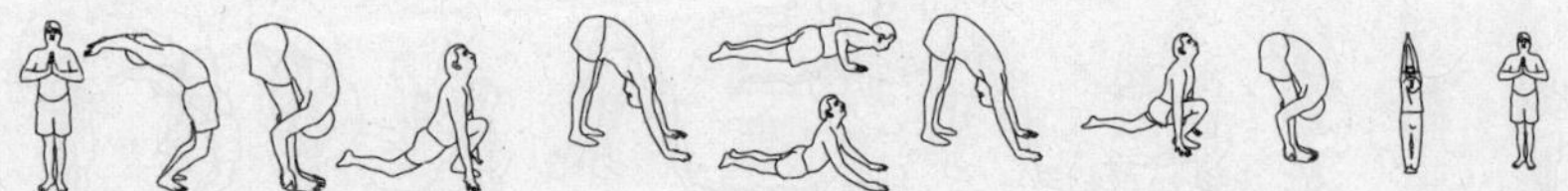

4. People with dark skin are less susceptible to the harmful effects of ultraviolet rays, whereas fair-skinned people are more prone to ultraviolet induced dangers. This is why more care is required for fairer people. Those who are albino (the people who lack melanin pigment in their skin) are at extreme risk of developing sun exposure induced hazards, so they should observe more caution.

5. In cloudy weather, only infrared radiation of the sun is reduced and not the ultraviolet radiation. This masks the heat sensation from the sunrays and thus increases the chances of ultraviolet induced injuries because of absence of any warning symptom.

6. Glass cabins are not good to prevent ultraviolet

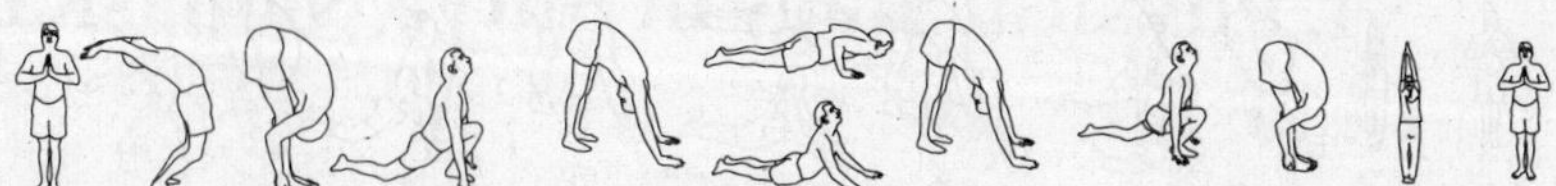

radiations and so precautions should also be taken when it is performed indoors where the sunrays enter through a glass partition.

7. Sun screens should be applied by people who are prone to sun burn.

In the normal practice of Surya Namaskar, the harmful effects of ultraviolet radiation are never observed because of the following reasons :

1. It takes very little time to finish the entire cycle of Surya Namaskar. Exposure to sunrays for such short periods even during midday does not cause any harmful effects on the body.

2. It is usually performed in the morning when the natural incidence of ultraviolet radiation is minimal.

4. Physical Stage of Surya Namaskar

Preparatory Phase

Preferably, do it outdoors to experience all the goodness of nature.

Wear light-coloured, loose clothes which can absorb less radiation and can leave you free to stretch your limbs to the extent possible.

Face the sun as you are going to receive the energy from it. It is imperative for the receiver to face the giver.

Practise on an even surface to avoid difficulties during the actual performance.

Place a carpet or clean bedsheet on the floor where this has to be practised so that earthly interferences are minimised.

Clean yourself before you start (empty the bowels and bladder).This is most important to give you a fresh feel both physically and mentally and will also enable you to perform to your highest capacity.

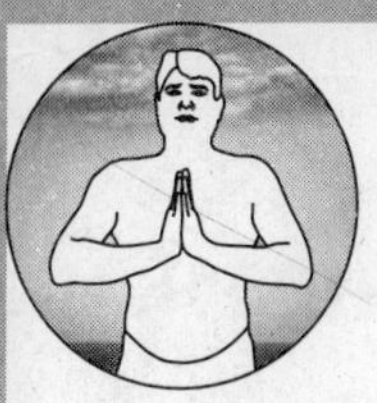

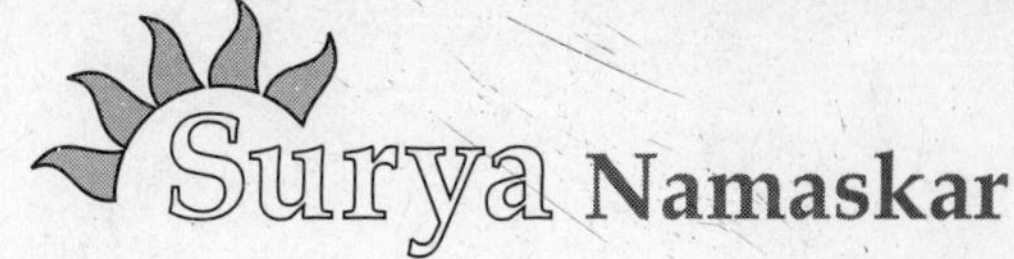

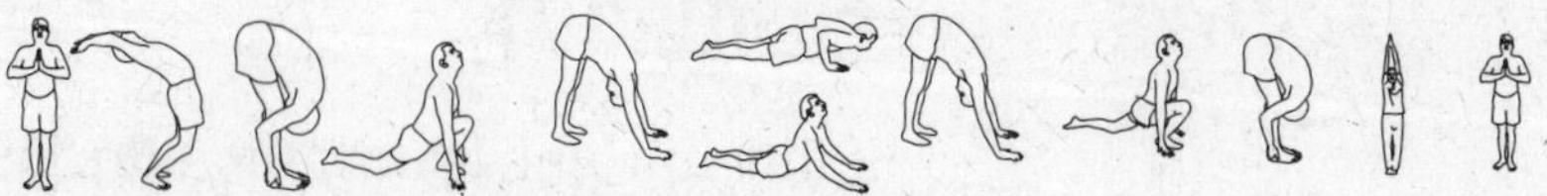

Relax completely to gain a full stretch. Any increase in muscle tone may interfere with the process of physical movements.

Feel receptive from within. This is probably the most important part of the preparatory phase. You will not be able to receive anything unless you are receptive.

You are now ready to receive from the largest energy reservoir of the universe.

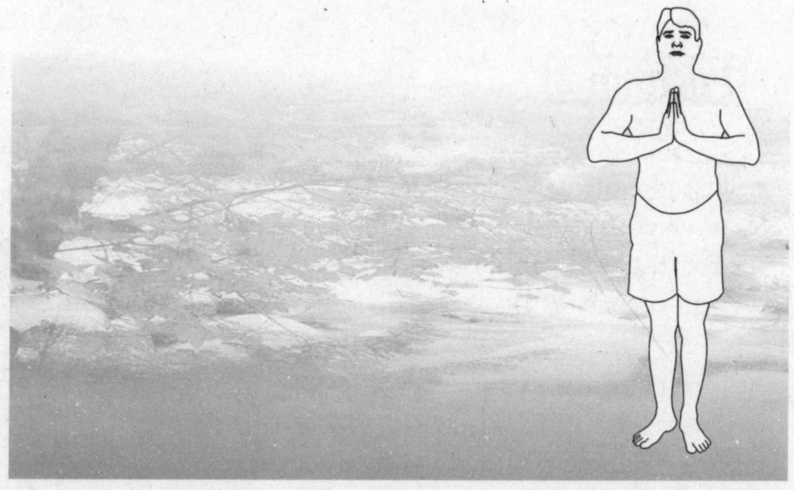

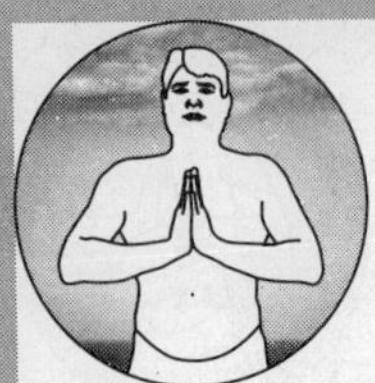

Surya Namaskar

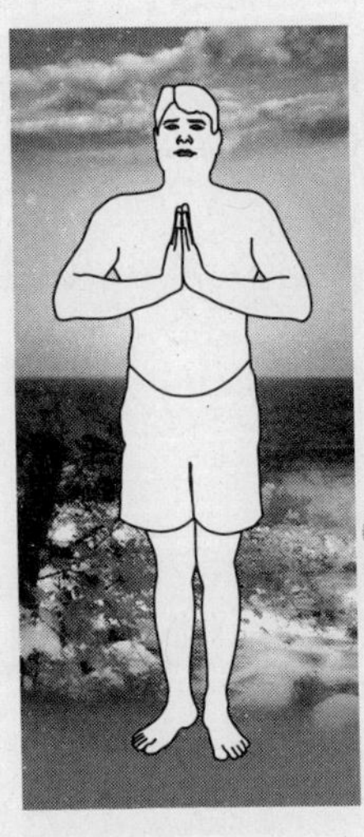

Position 1

- Stand upright facing the sun Feel completely relaxed.
- Place the lower limbs slightly apart.
- Put your weight equally on both limbs Feel as though you are beginning the divine dance to salute Nature.
- Bring your hands towards your chest and join your palms in a namaste.

Position 2

- Start elevating your arms above your head.
- Keep them straight above your head with palms towards the sun.
- Start bending posteriorly to the extent possible with folded hands.

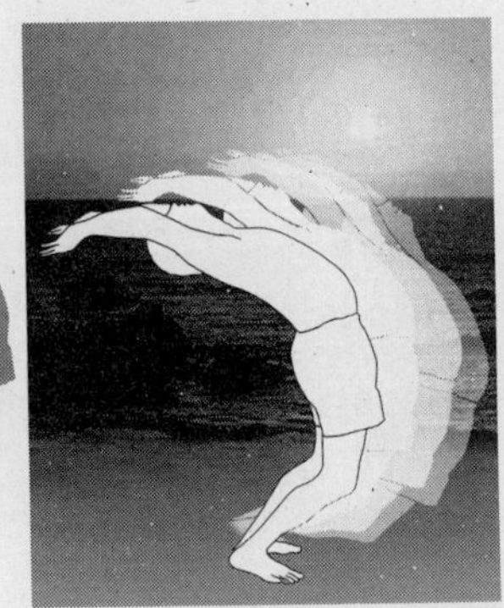

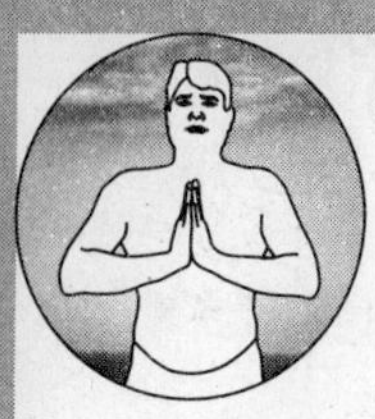

Surya Namaskar

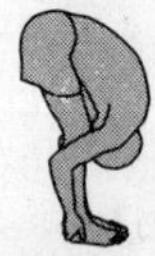

Position 3

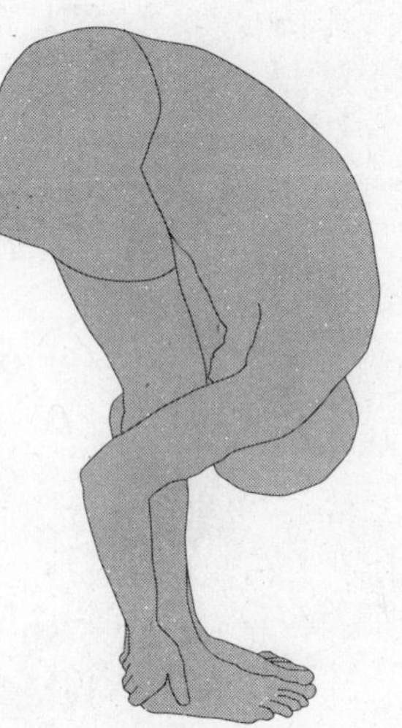

- Come forward to stand straight in an upright position.
- Start bending down from the lumber spine.
- Bring your head down to your toes with your fingers.
- Keep the knee straight during the entire process.

Position 4

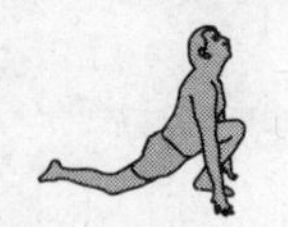

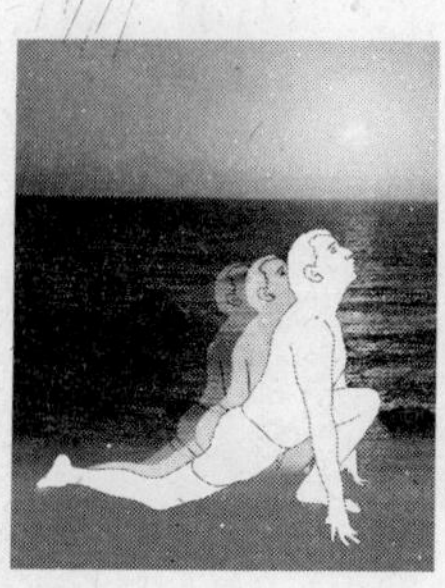

- Place your palms on the ground.
- Stretch your left leg back to the extent possible.
- Place your left too on the ground.
- Bend the right leg forward.
- Push the waist downward.
- Push your shoulders up and backwards.
- Push your shoulder up and backwards.
- Stretch your head backwards.
- Try to see the sky with your eyes facing upward.

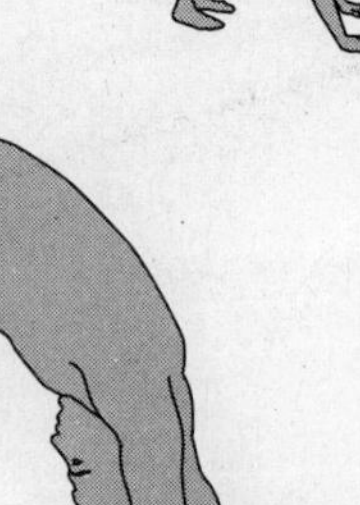

Position 5

- Bring your right leg back to the ground.
- Keep your right toe on the ground.
- Keep the weight of your body on both hands.
- Push your chest down and forward.
- Push your shoulder downward.
- Push your hips upward.

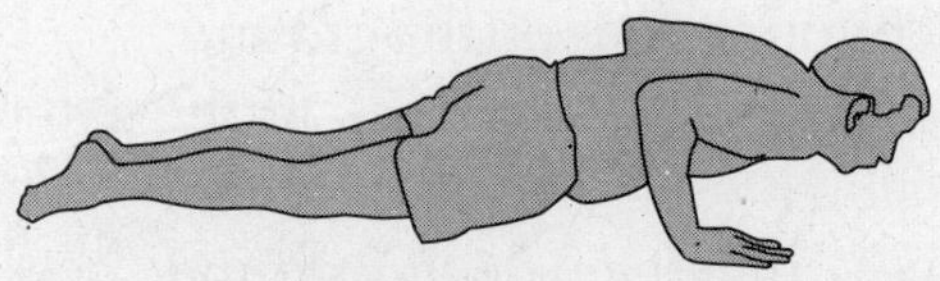

Position 6

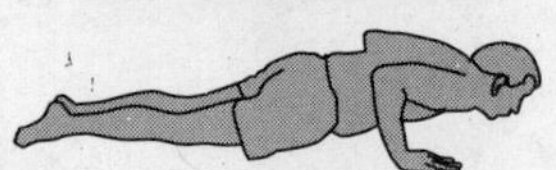

- Stand upright facing the sun.
- Feel completely relaxed.
- Place the lower limbs slightly apart.
- Put your weight equally on both limbs.
- Feel as though you are beginning the divine dance to salute Nature.
- Bring your hands towards your chest and join your palms in a namaste.

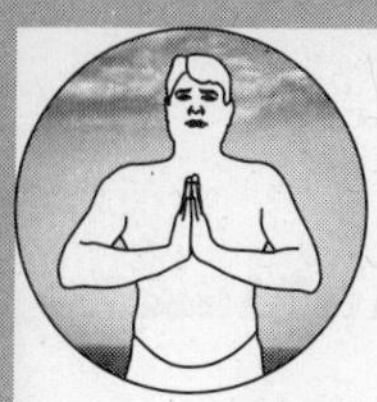

Surya Namaskar

Position 7

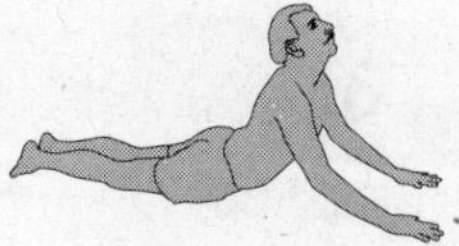

- Straighten your arms.
- Push your chest forward.
- Bend the head back to face up.
- Relax your waist completely.
- Stretch it downwards.

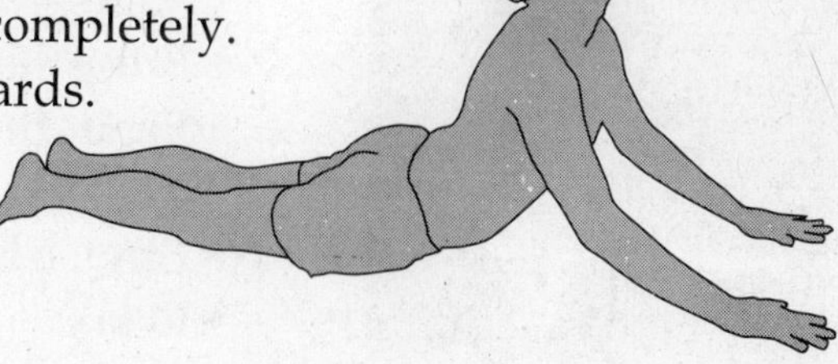

Position 8

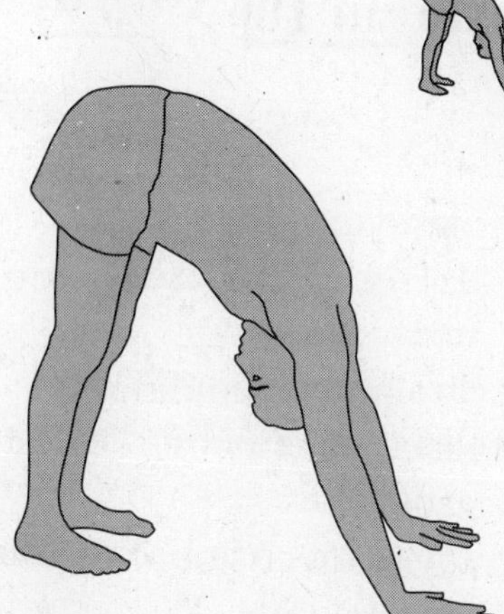

- Shift the centre of gravity by placing your weight on your feet.
- Swing back.
- Push your hips upward.
- Push your chest downward.
- Keep your head pointing down.
- Look at your navel.

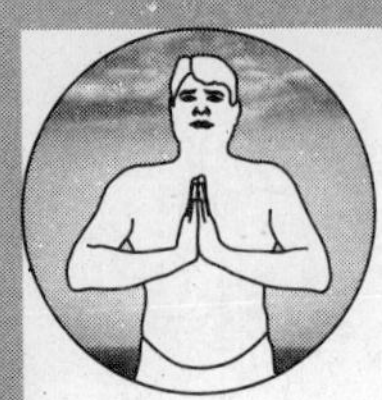

Position 9

- Transfer your weight to your hands.
- Thrust your chest upwards.
- Keep your head facing up.
- Try to look upwards by straining your cervical spine.
- Bring the right leg forward.
- Bend the right leg at the knee.
- Stretch backwards.
- Relax.

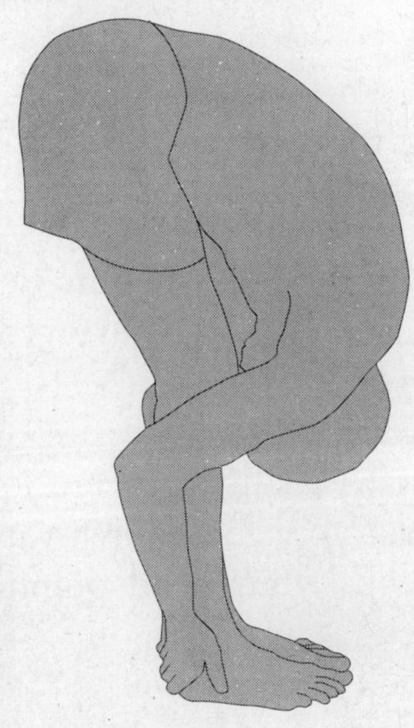

Position 10

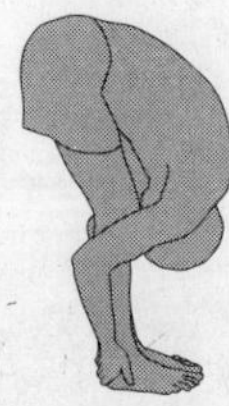

- Stand upright.
- Bring your left leg forward.
- Straighten your knees.
- Place your palms on the ground.
- Try to touch your head to your knees.

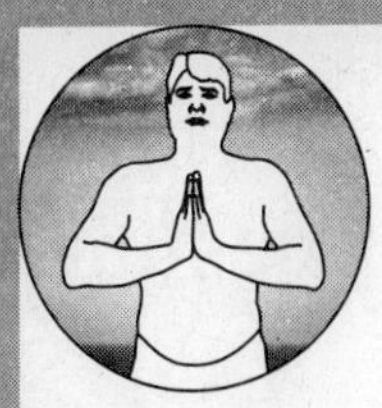

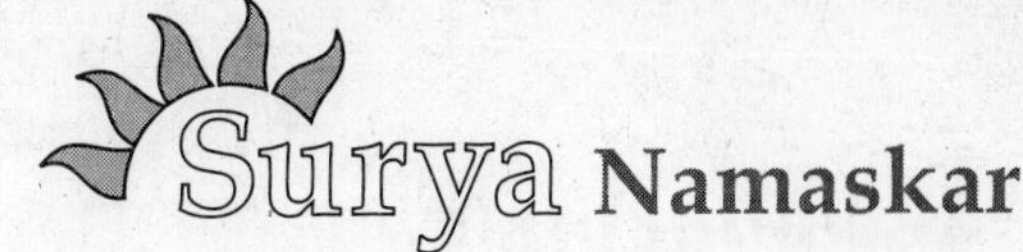

Surya Namaskar

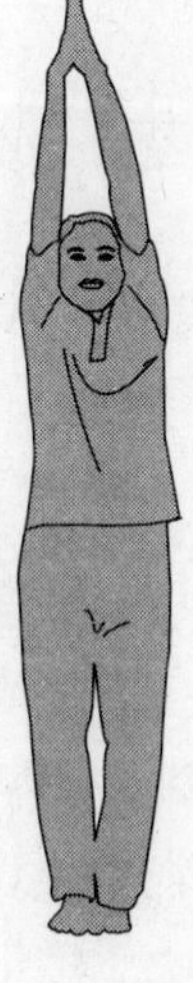

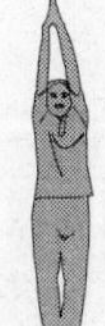

Position 11

- Stand upright slowly.
- Stretch backwards as much as possible.

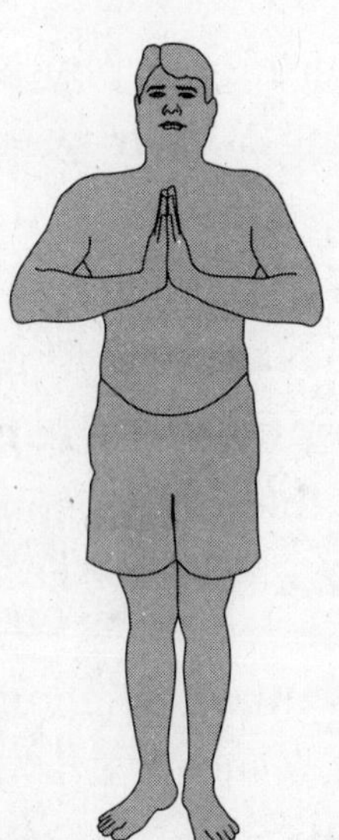

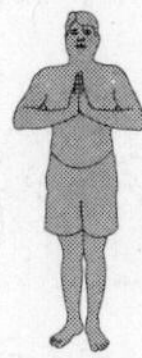

Position 12

- Stand upright slowly.
- Join your palms in a namaste as done at the start.
- Relax yourself completely.

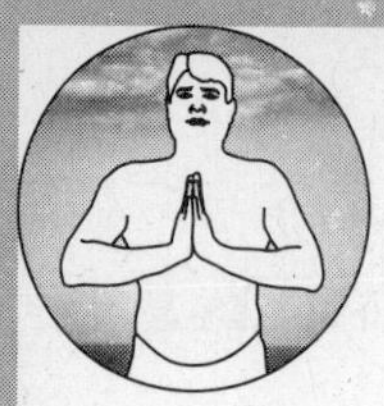

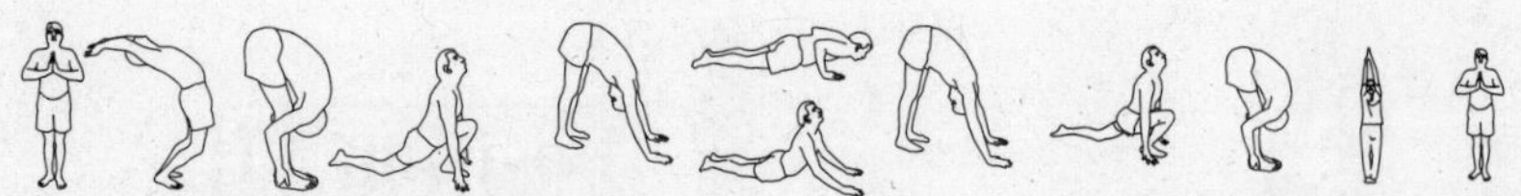

This completes one set of Surya Namaskar. The next set should be started by bending the left leg first in position 4. A complete set usually takes one to two minutes. However, for beginners, it is prudent to spend more time so that the stress points can be well understood during the actual movements. Four to eight sets can be performed at a time and this largely depends upon the individual's capacity and condition. The onset of sweating indicates that you should stop the exercises for the moment. The most important things to remember during the physical phase of Surya Namaskar are the shifting of your weight from arms to legs and from legs to arms and relaxation/stretch at the specific parts of the spine. The essence of the physical part of Surya Namaskar is the alternative forward and backward bending of different segments of the spine which makes the whole spine, flexible.

The physical part of Surya Namaskar should essentially be followed by relaxation. Corpus posture *(shavasana)* is the best way of physical relaxation. The body

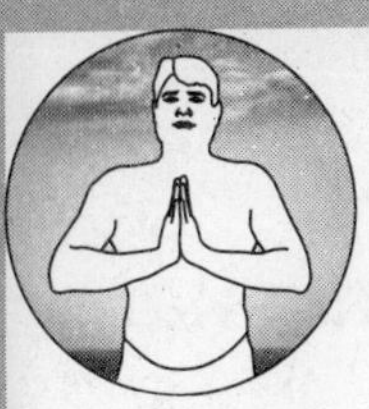

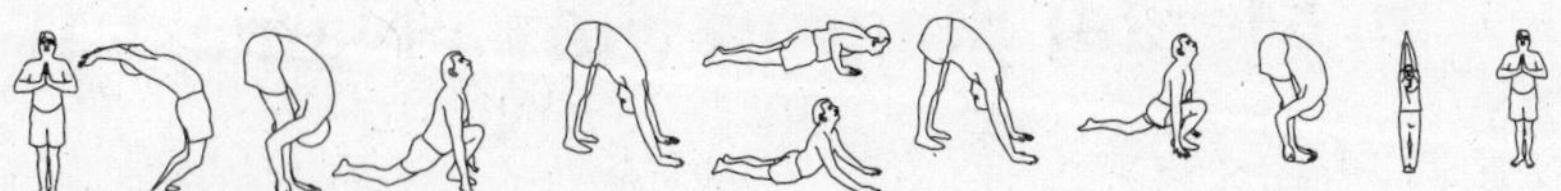

should be stretched initially with exaggerated tones and then gradually relaxed. This gives complete relaxation to the muscles which are tired due to overuse.

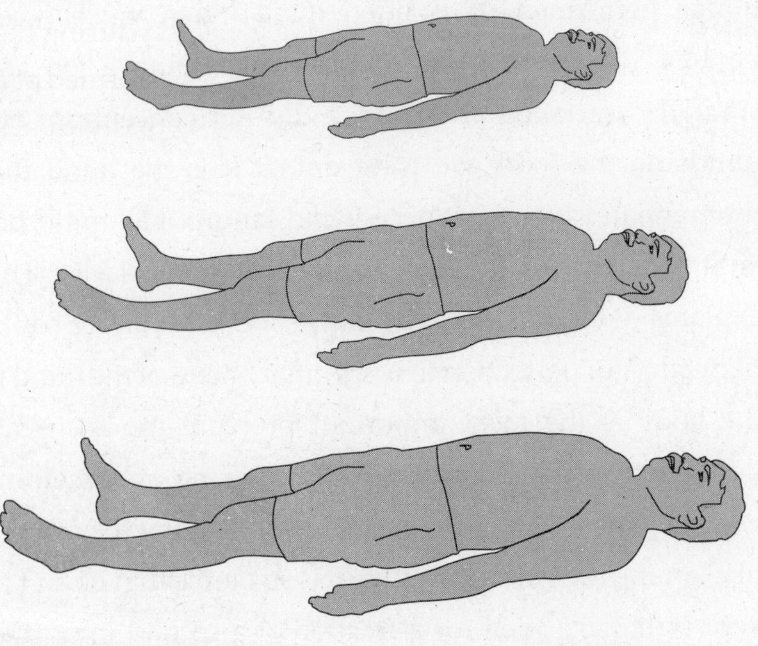

Shavasana

5. Mental Stage of Surya Namaskar

Breathing has been the favourite tool of sages from time immemorial to tame the mind. The mind is the single most important factor to determine the net outcome of things performed. It is often quoted that we succeed because we applied our minds while doing a job and similarly we failed because we did not concentrate our minds on the work we were doing. It is the mind that differentiates between success and failure. The mind has an inherent characteristic of unity and molecularity. This explains why at one time only one job can be done perfectly. For perfection in work, attachment of the mind to the body is the most important prerequisite. So, while doing something if your mind is thinking of something else, perfection can never be achieved. Taming the mind is like taming the wildest animal. It is so motile that it can't be kept stationary even for a fraction of a second in normal conditions. The best way to tame the mind is to keep it engaged in something. Do you remember the old story of a

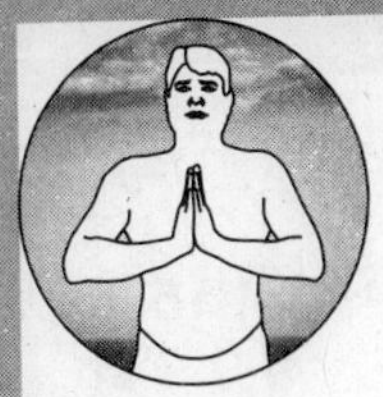

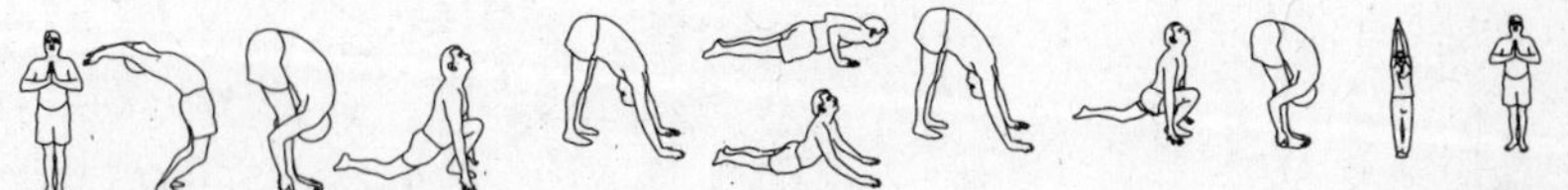

devil who repeatedly asked for a job threatening that he would eat his own master otherwise? After getting tired of assigning him jobs, the master thought of a trick as there were no more jobs to give. He assigned him the jobs of climbing up and getting down a pole repeatedly. The devil was busy and the master was free. To concentrate upon breathing is the trick to tame this devil, the mind. This is one of the most obvious, vital and continuous processes where even the most motile substance can be engaged.

In Surya Namaskar this breathing phenomenon is beautifully amalgamated with the physical rhythms, which give rise to a unique dynamic meditation.

Breathing in the normal course is an involuntary process and constitutes two basic components. These are inhalation and exhalation.

Inhalation, where the air is taken in, is an active process and requires consumption of energy to take the air

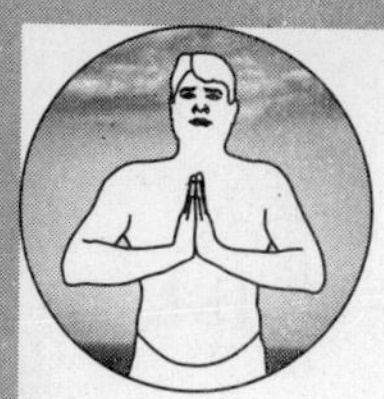

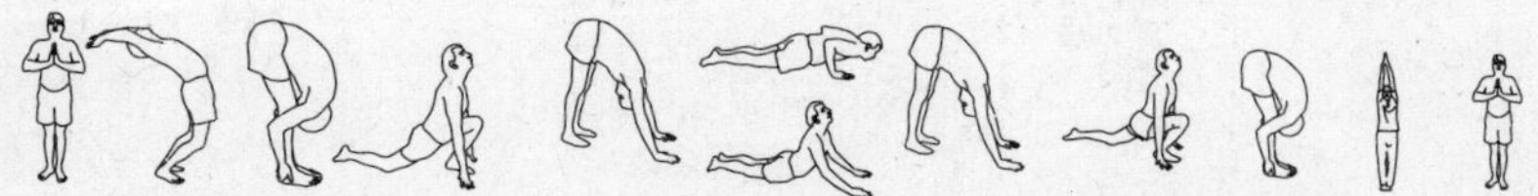

inside the respiratory tract. On the contrary, exhalation is a passive process and does not require any expenditure of energy. Pranayama or the breathing regulatory exercises are the processes to control the breathing process voluntarily. Now, as in Surya Namaskar there are certain rhythmic postures which are done voluntarily, for voluntary breathing, the best is when we are static. In Surya Namaskar, inhalation is usually done at the time of static postures or during the backward bending movements and exhalation is done at the time of the active forward bending movements. The reasons are obvious. When we are engaged in one voluntary activity, it is not possible to do another voluntary activity at the same time and so the only time for breathing in, is when we are static. The other reason for doing the inhalations during posterior bending and exhalation during forward bending is also simple. When we bend forward, the abdomen is being pressed. This increases the intra-abdominal pressure and makes the movement of the diaphragm difficult. As the

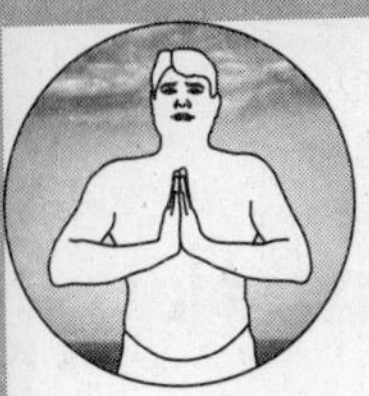

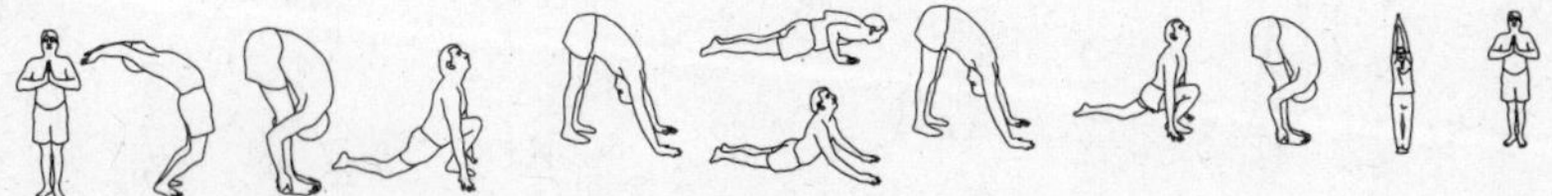

process of inhalation essentially involves the movement of the diaphragm, the process of breathing in also becomes difficult. In the process of backward bending, the situation is reversed and this makes inhalation easier.

By keeping a voluntary control over breathing, the whole process of Surya Namaskar comes under voluntary control and this is how the mind is tamed. The mind is tamed in Surya Namaskar because we keep it engaged for the whole process. As it is not left unattended at any time, the chances of it deviating are minimal.

The breathing regulatory activities associated with different positions of salutation are these:

Position 1

Stand upright facing the sun

Feel completely relaxed

Place the lower limbs slightly apart

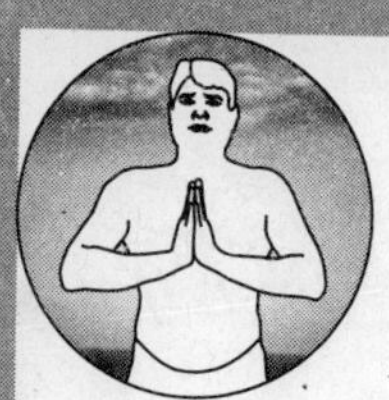

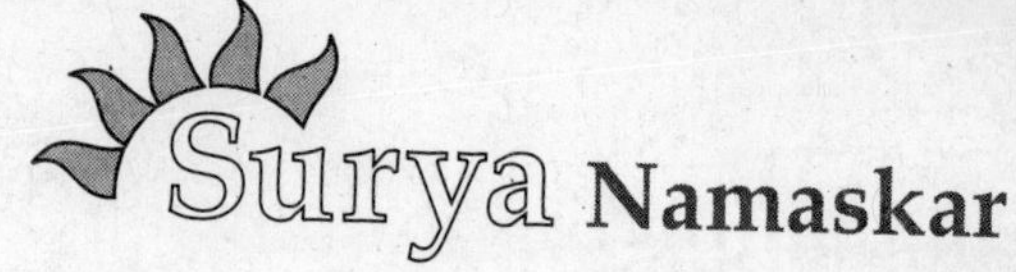

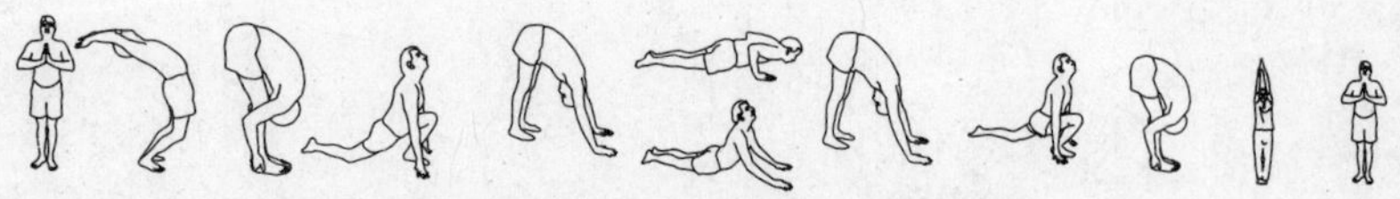

Put your weight equally on both limbs

Feel as though you are beginning the divine dance to salute nature

Bring your hands towards your chest and join your palms in a *namaste*

Position 2

Start elevating your arms above your head

Keep them straight above your head with palms towards the sun

Start bending posteriorly to the extent possible with folded hands

Position 3

Come forward to stand straight in an upright position

Start bending down from the lumber spine

Bring your head down to your knees

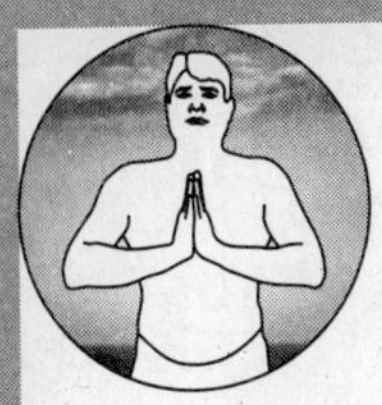

Surya Namaskar

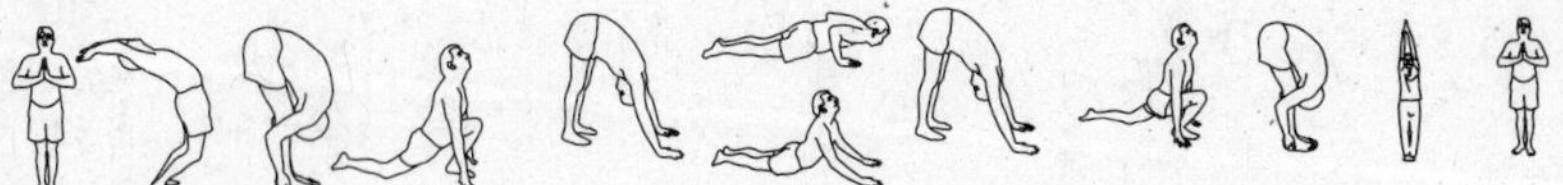

Touch your toes with your fingers

Keep the knee straight during the entire process

Position 4

Place your palms on the ground

Stretch your left leg back to the extent possible

Place your left toe on the ground

Bend the right leg forward

Push the waist downward

Push your shoulders up and backwards

Stretch your head backwards

Try to see the sky with your eyes facing upward

Position 5

Bring your right leg back to the ground

Keep your right toe on the ground

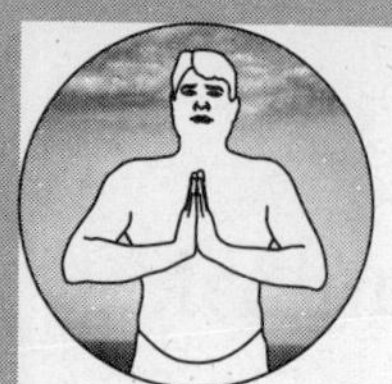

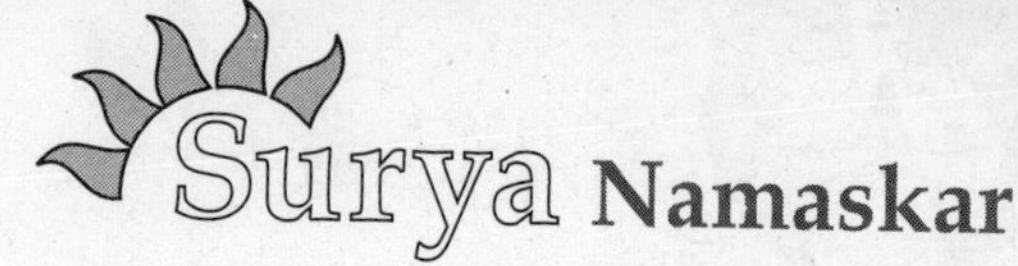

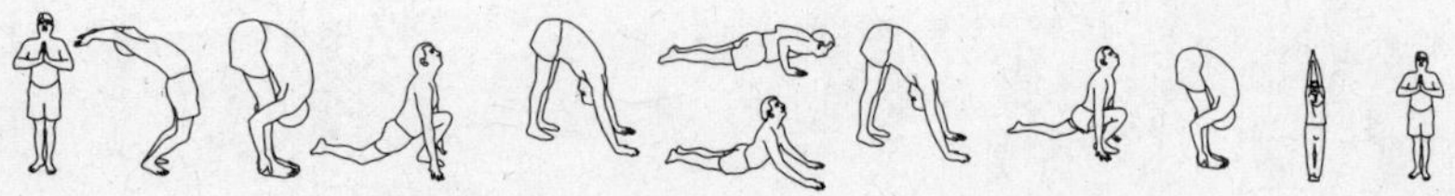

Keep the weight of your body on both hands

Push your chest down and forward

Push your shoulder downward

Push your hips upward

Push your head inwards

Try to see your navel by turning your eyes towards it

Position 6

Bring your head up

Start looking in front by facing forward

Shift the weight of your body on to your hands

Fold your arms to get down to the ground

Keep your body a little away from the ground

Swing forward on your hands

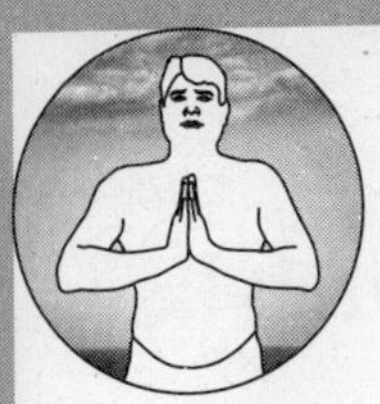

Surya Namaskar

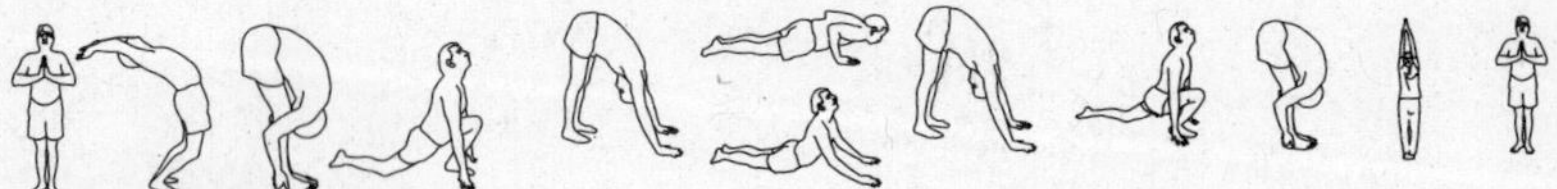

Position 7

Straighten your arms

Push your chest forward

Bend the head back to face up

Relax your waist completely

Stretch it downwards

Position 8

Shift the centre of gravity by placing your weight on your feet

Swing back

Push your hips upward

Push your chest downward

Keep your head pointing down

Look at your navel

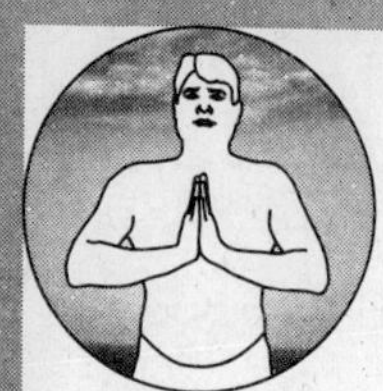

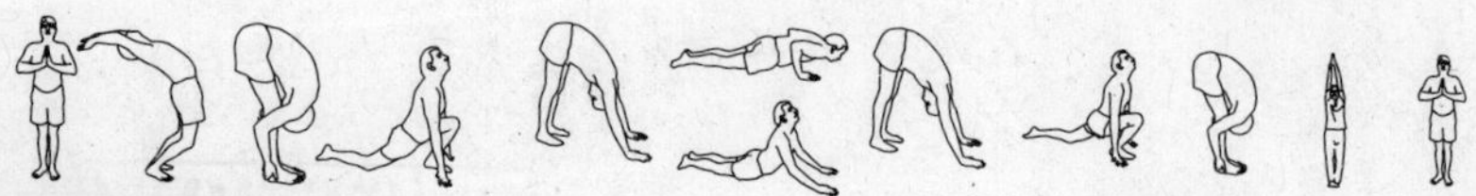

Position 9

Transfer your weight to your hands

Thrust your chest upwards

Keep your head facing up

Try to look upwards by straining your cervical spine

Bring the right leg forward

Bend the right leg at the knee

Stretch backwards

Relax

Position 10

Stand upright

Bring your left leg forward

Straighten your knees

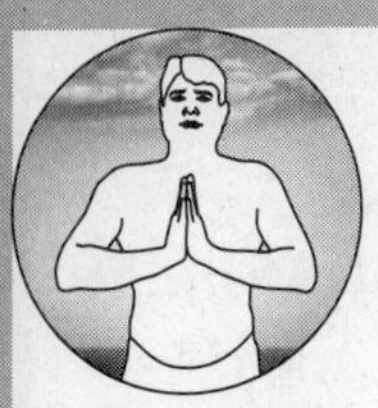

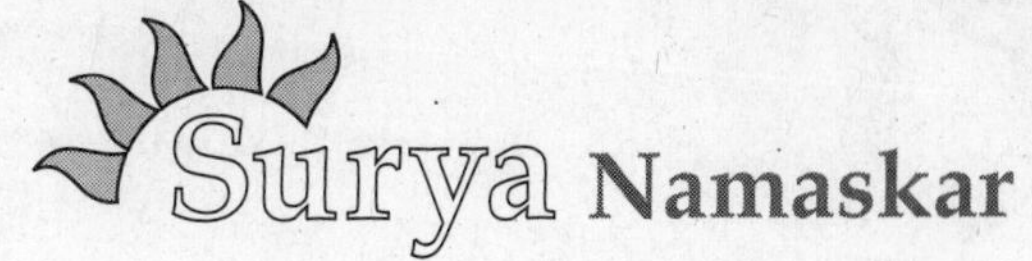

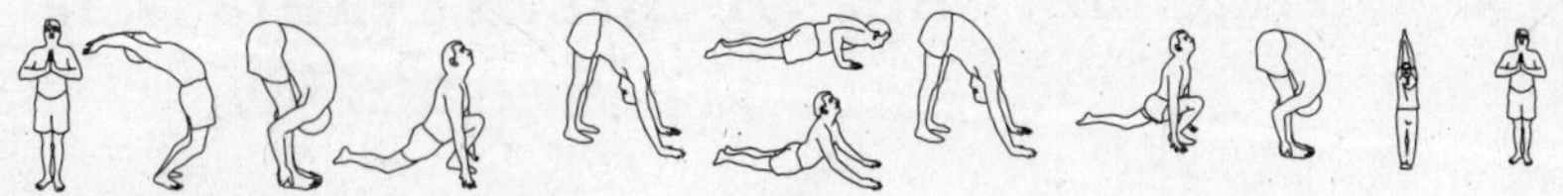

Place your palms on the ground

Try to touch your head to your knees

Position 11

Stand upright slowly

Stretch backwards as much as possible

Position 12

Stand upright slowly

Join your palms in a *namaste* as done at the start

Relax yourself completely

The next set of salutation can be started just after a few normal breaths.

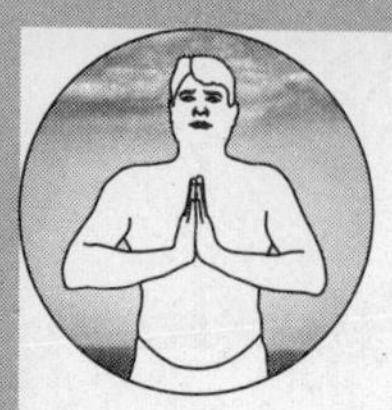

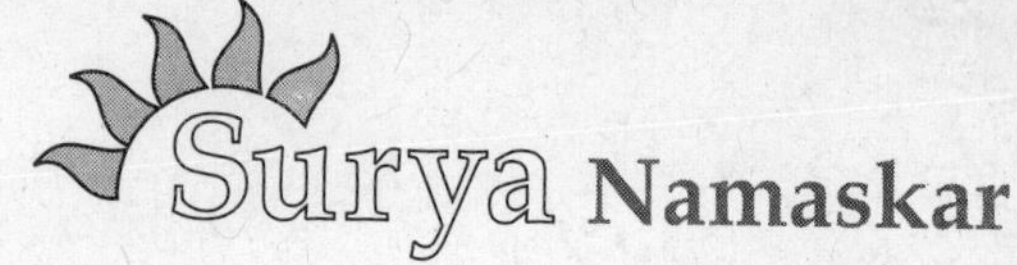

6. Spiritual Stage of Surya Namaskar

The spiritual stage of Surya Namaskar is the combination of the physical and mental components to achieve the spiritual goal. At this stage, with each set of exercises is added the recitation of a *bija* mantra which praises the sun for its different activities through which it blesses the world. These mantras are to be uttered silently in the mind and with complete devotion to the deity to which it is offered.

Every mantra starts with OM which is the initiating mantra (Pranava mantra). OM represents the supreme deity which is non-dual. Every mantra has a presiding deity. The belief is that when one chants a mantra, with the mental visualisation of the deity for whom the mantra is chanted, it creates a link between the energies of the man and the power. Now as a rule, energy flows in the direction where it is deficient. Naturally we receive the positive energy from the deity to whom we are praying. The mantras to be chanted with the physical steps are the following :

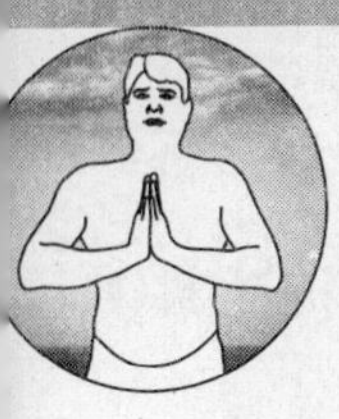

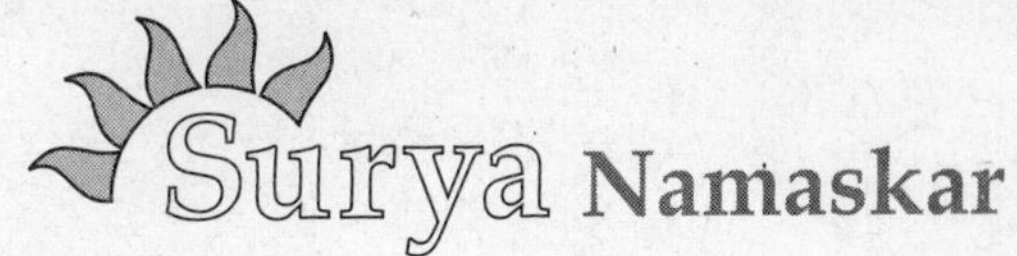

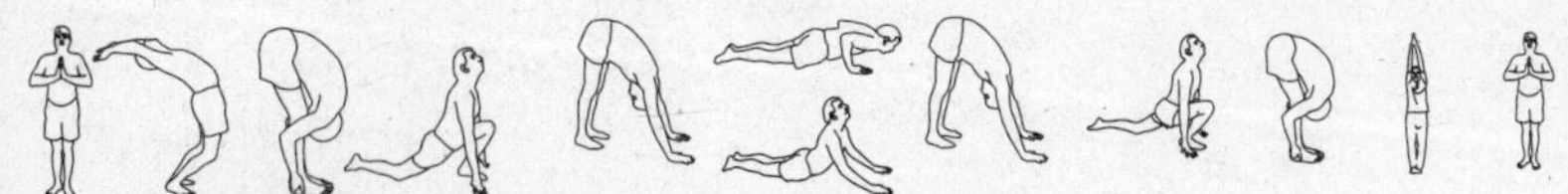

Position 1

Om Mitraya Namah

Medyati snehayati iti mitrah

This is the Sanskrit derivation for Mitra who causes *snehana* (oleation) and *medana* (nourishment).

This is the mantra chanted in praise of the mitra (mitra= friendly) nature of the sun through which life becomes possible. It is a known fact that the very existence of life on earth is possible only because of the sun which gives essential energy to green plants and enables them to carry out photosynthesis. This photosynthesis in a broader perspective becomes the basis of the food pyramid. Praying this mantra can give us strength to become friendly with everyone, as the sun is with the universe.

Position 2

Om Suryaya Namaha

Suvati karmani lokam preryati va

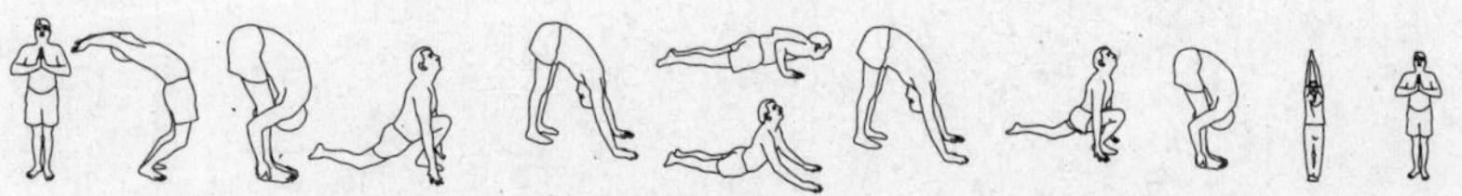

This is the Sanskrit derivation for the word *Surya*. The one who stimulates the world to start anything is called *Surya*. *Surya* hallmarks the beginning of the day and naturally stimulates the beginning of all activities which are essential for life. This mantra is chanted in praise of the stimulant nature of *Surya* and praying this mantra can give us the strength to become the stimulator of various activities for people around us.

Position 3

Om Ravaye Namah

Ruyate stuyate iti ravi

The one who is worshipped because of its uncountable blessings is called Ravi. This mantra is recited in praise of Ravi who earmarks the supportive nature of the sun. By praying this mantra, we can become as respectable as the sun is by having similar characteristics that the sun has.

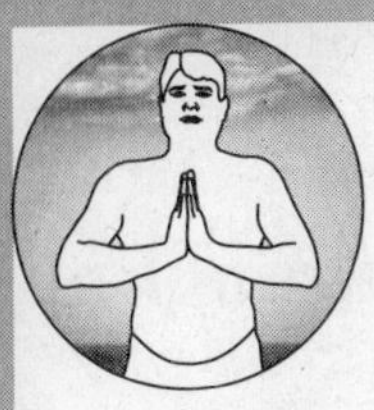

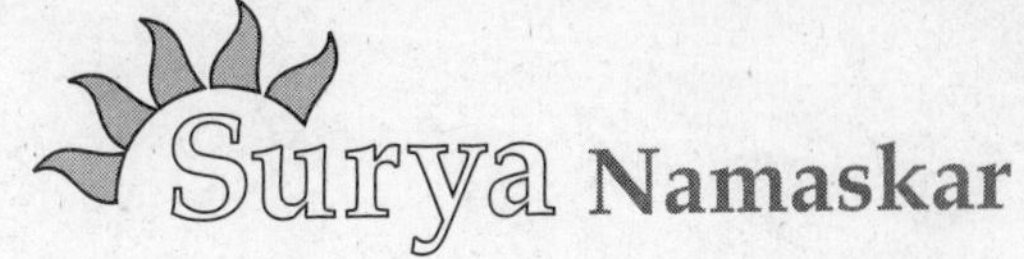

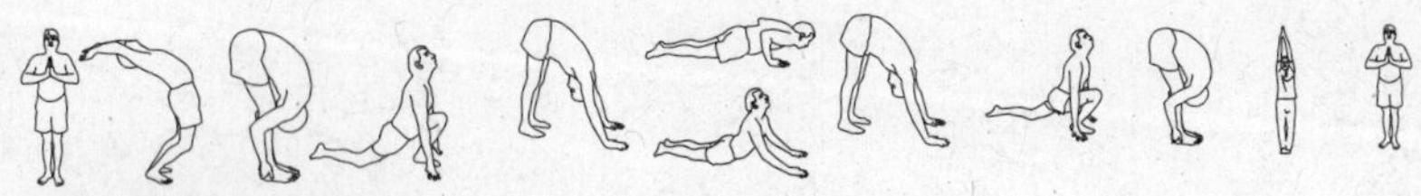

Position 4

Om Bhanve Namah

Bhati chaturdasha bhuvneshu swa prabhaya deeptaye iti bhanu

The one who not only is himself illuminated, but also illuminates the whole world is called Bhanu. This mantra is in praise of the bhanu nature of the sun which asks for self-illumination first and then to illuminate others who are around us. This may be the most beautiful of all qualities that a man can have. By praying this mantra, we can become enlightened and once we are enlightened, the others around us are sure to be illuminated.

Position 5

Om Khagaya Namah

Khe nabhasi gacchati iti khaga

The one whose passage is sky is called Khaga.

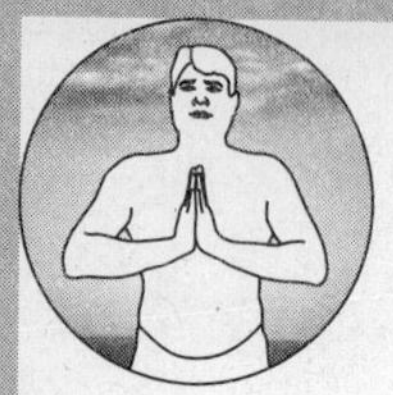

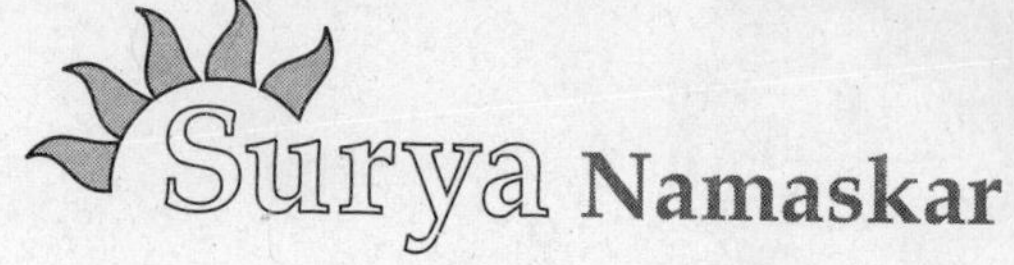

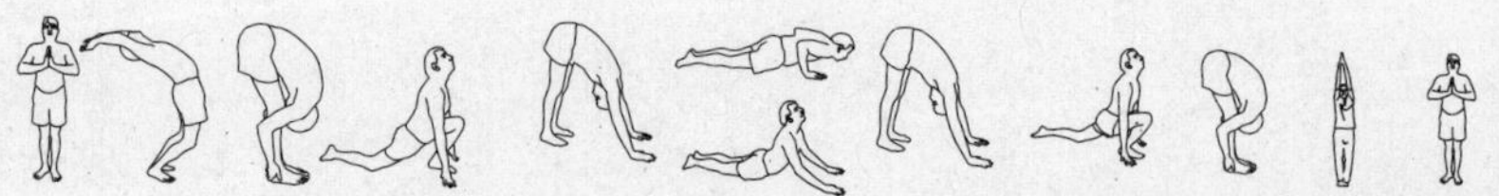

This is the mantra recited in praise of Khaga (Kha= sky, Ga=one which moves in). The sun is the only object in the sky which moves (at least empirically as it seems from earth) to cause day and night. And, moreover, it is eternal. This is the only eternal object in the sky. Praying this mantra can give us the strength to be as stable as the sun is in the sky.

Position 6

Om Pushnaye Namah

Push vraddho

The one who helps to increase strength is called pushana. The sun is helpful in providing nutrition to the earth in many direct and indirect ways. The most important characteristic is that it is prolife. It supports the very existence of life on earth. Praying this mantra imbibes us with the energy that supports life and provides a positive environment which supports the growth and sustenance of life.

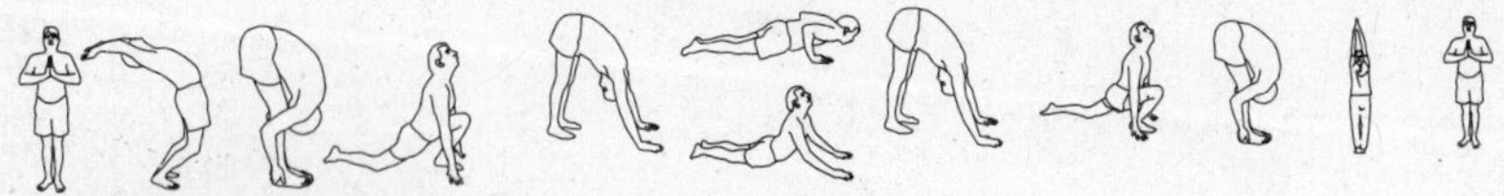

Position 7

Om Hiranya Garbhaye Namah

Hiranyam hemmayandam garbha utpatti sthanam asya

The one whose central part is as bright as gold and which is the progenitor of everything is called hiranyagarbha. Be as bright as gold and be as fertile as the sun. This is the essence of being hiranyagarbha. The literal meaning is that as the inside of the sun is like gold, you also become pure as gold from inside.

Position 8

Om Marichyaye Namah

Mriyante nashyanti chudra jantava tamansi va

The one whose mere presence is capable of eradicating darkness and also the things which flourish in darkness, is called Marich. Be as bright as the sun so all the darkness from inside and around cannot exist. This darkness is not

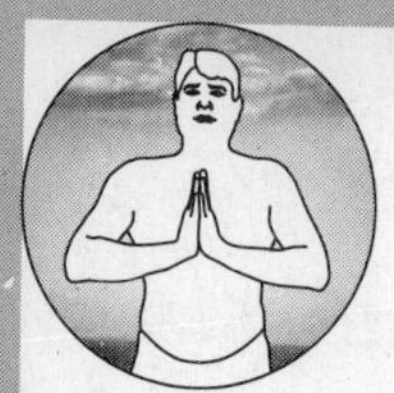

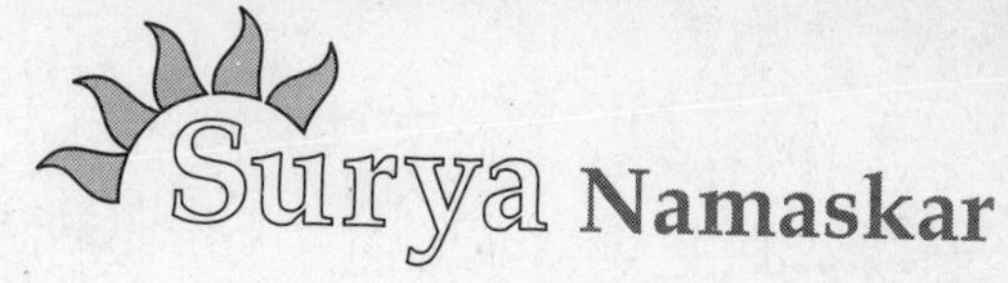

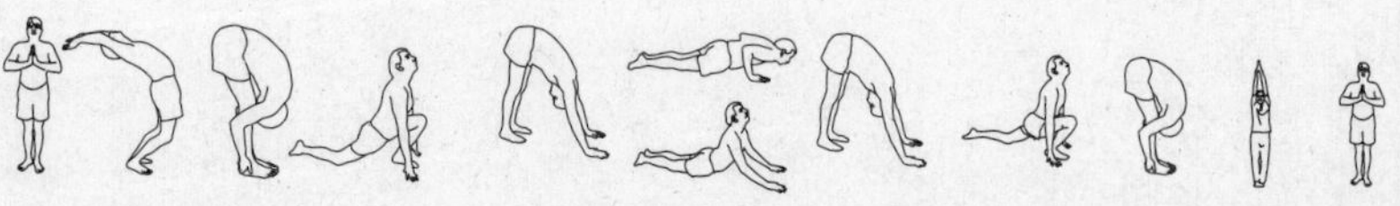

only physical darkness but also the darkness of the mind and the things which flourish in darkness. Various disease-causing pathogens require lower ambient temperature and darkness for their growth and survival. The ultraviolet component of the sun's radiation is capable of eradicating these pathogens. Praying this mantra gives one the quality of eradicating darkness and its effects from all around.

Position 9

Om Aadityaya Namah

Aditi apatyam adityaya iti

The one who is born of Aditi is Aditya. This mantra is prayed in praise of Aditya.

Position 10

Om Savitrai Namah

Sarva loka prasavnat savita iti prakirtite

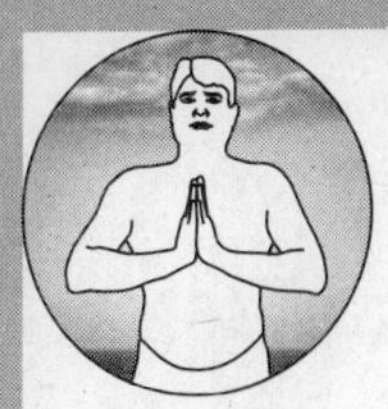

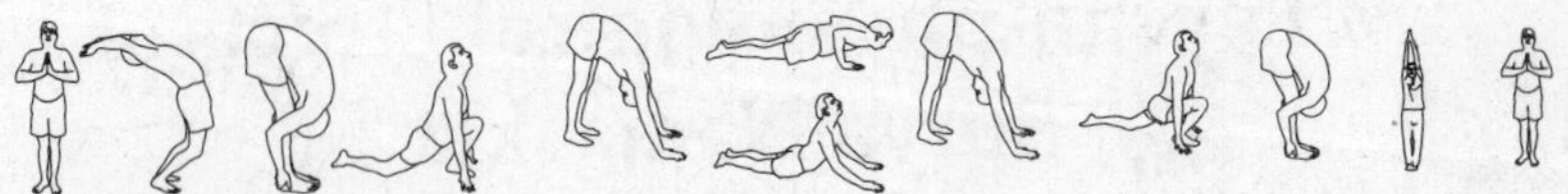

One who has given birth to the whole universe is called Savita. It exemplifies the quality of the sun for taking on pain and giving life to the earth. It is known that the sun produces energy and light through atomic fusion and as this process has continued since time immemorial, the sun is losing weight and is shrinking. This mantra prays for the quality of the sun as a pain-bearer to give birth to a new life.

Position 11

Om Arkaya Namah

The one who is worshipped because of its qualities is called Arka. This worship is done to gain the qualities of the sun so that one can be known for one's qualities.

Position 12

Om Bhaskaraya Namah

Bhasam karoti iti bhaskara:

The one who is illuminated is called Bhaskara. This is the prayer to become as illuminated as the sun.

7. Psycho-physiological Effects of Surya Namaskar

Is yoga enough to keep you fit? Bauman Alisa in an article published in Yoga Journal, Sept./Oct. 2002 has beautifully elaborated the physiological principles involved in the practice of yoga, which are supposed to keep a person fit by practising it on a regular basis. A comparison of muscle strength, endurance, flexibility and lung capacity between yoga practitioners and the top performers of different sports has been made and this has revealed some of the most outstanding results. A university sports medicine lab [at the University of California at Davis] was given the task of testing three yogis for strength, endurance, flexibility and lung capacity and concluded as follows:

Flexibility: The yogis compare favourably with top performers who train for maximum flexibility in fields like gymnastics and ballet.

Body composition: According to skin fold measurements taken with calipers, all three yogis had

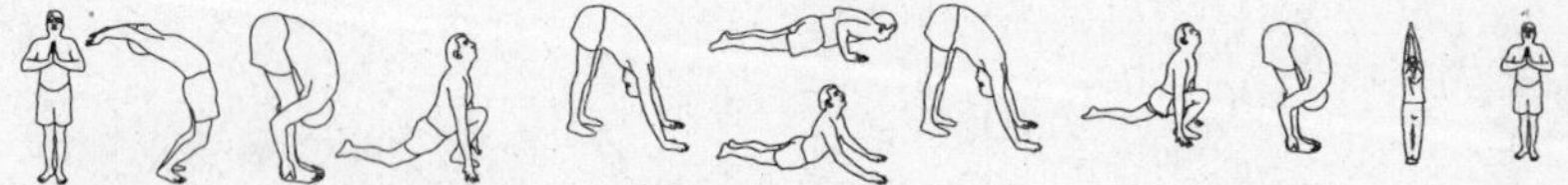

body fat ratios and body mass indices comparable to those of elite endurance athletes like top marathoners and cyclists.

Muscular strength, endurance and balance: Based on biodex tests on elbow and knee flexion and extension, measuring maximum force exerted, muscle endurance and muscle balance – both between the right and left sides and between agonist and antagonist muscles – the yogis scored mostly within or near normal ranges.

Lung capacity: Using a spirometer, two of the yogis performed within a few percentage points of the norm and one performed better than the norm.

Cardio-respiratory fitness: All three yogis produced the O_2 maximum measurements in the same range as fairly active athletes did.

The results documented in this study linked every

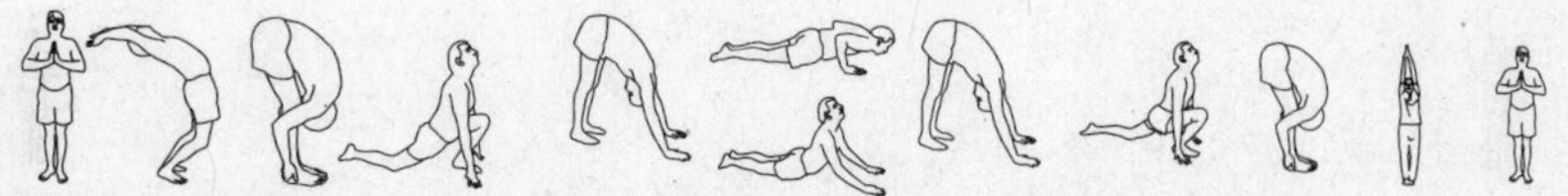

physiological benefit associated with active sport with that of yoga practice. These results match beautifully with the first stage of Surya Namaskar, where stress is laid on the rhythmic physical activities of the body. People who don't want to reach a higher stage of Surya Namaskar can be sufficiently benefitted with the physical aspect of the exercises involved in Surya Namaskar.

Substantial research has been made to evaluate yoga on contemporary scientific parameters. Surya Namaskar has not been experimented on in isolation to prove its worth to the world in the way yoga has been, but still, as Surya Namaskar essentially involves the core of yoga practices including the asana, the pranayama and the chanting of mantras, it is bound to have the same effects as routine yoga practices.

The addition of the chanting of mantras to Surya Namaskar also causes beneficial physiological and psychological effects as is concluded in a recent research

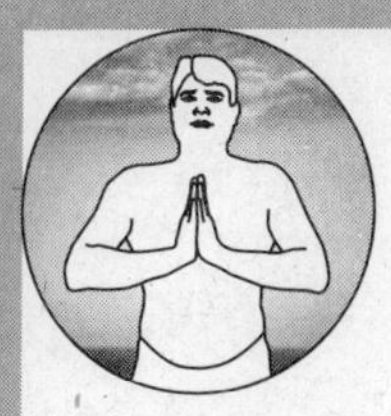

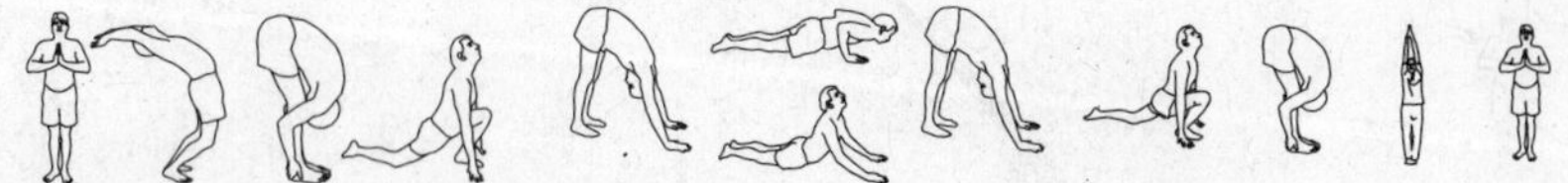

published in the British Medical Journal (Bernardi *et. al.* 2001). They have tried to identify the effect of the rosary prayers and yoga mantras on autonomic cardiovascular rhythms in a comparative study. The objective of the study was to test whether rhythmic formulae such as the rosary and yoga mantras can synchronise and reinforce inherent cardiovascular rhythms and modify baroreflex sensitivity. A comparison of effects of the recitation of the Ave Maria (in Latin) or of a mantra, during spontaneous and metronome controlled breathing, on breathing rate and on spontaneous oscillations in RR interval, and on blood pressure and cerebral circulation, was made and evaluated in twenty-three healthy adults. The main features taken for comparison were breathing rate, regularity of breathing, baroreflex sensitivity and frequency of cardiovascular oscillations. The results of the study have shown both prayer and mantra caused striking, powerful and synchronous increases in existing cardiovascular rhythms when recited six times a minute. Baroreflex sensitivity also

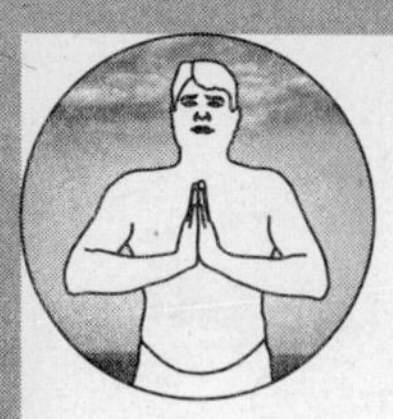

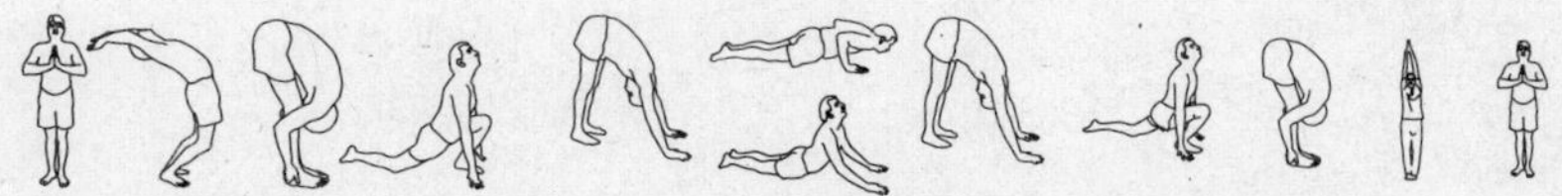

increased significantly and this could induce favourable psychological and possibly physiological effects.

A ten-week pilot study to evaluate the therapeutic benefits of yoga has been done by Czamara, Joli Michele (2002). The purpose of this study was to determine whether a ten-week yoga practice of postures, breathing and relaxation can increase a person's strength, balance, functional flexibility and the mental and physical qualities of life. Sixteen volunteers were recruited from a community-based yoga centre in New York. A quasi-experimental, one-group within subject control, pre-post-test design was used for this study. Data was analysed at the end and the study suggests that even a relatively short (ten-week) programme of yoga results in improvements of lower limb strength and the self-perception of the mental well-being of community-dwelling adults (mean age = 46.81), who are novice yoga practitioners. Research done at the Defence Institute of Physiology and Allied Sciences, Delhi, India

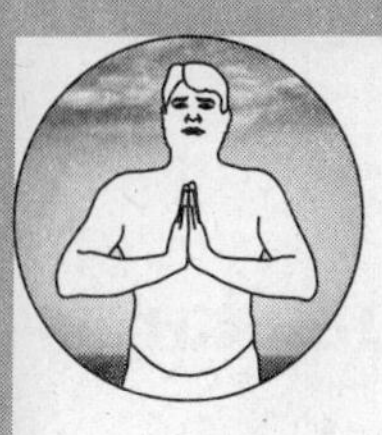

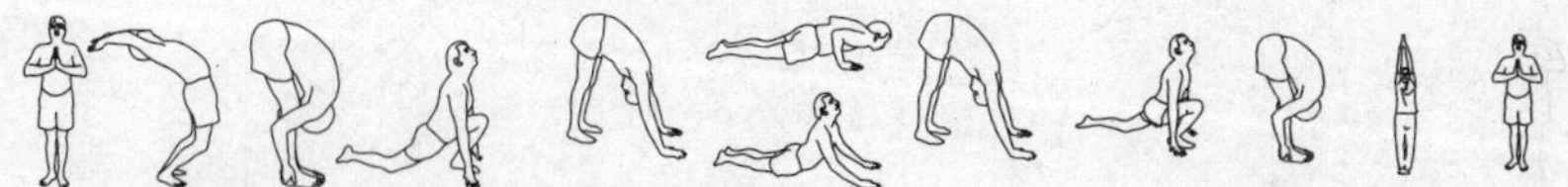

has tried to define the effect of yogic practices on the physiological and antioxidant systems in man. Under this study, maximal oxygen consumption and anaerobic threshold were determined on forty army subjects. They were divided into two groups, i.e. "yoga" and "control." The yoga group underwent one hour of yogic practices, consisting of asanas, pranayama, and meditation, every day except Sunday for twelve months. During this period, recordings were repeated in the seventh to eighth months and the twelfth to fourteenth months. During each exercise session on a bicycle ergometer, blood samples were taken before and after exhaustive exercise to assess the subject's level of oxidative stress due to exercise, by recording various markers of oxidative stress and antioxidant activity to observe if there is any effect of yogic practices in the modulation of oxidative stress. Tests were conducted on twenty yoga proficient participants (yoga instructors) for recording of various physiological parameters during yogic practices. Among them eight subjects showed better

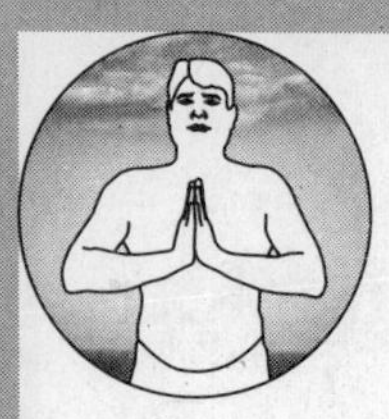

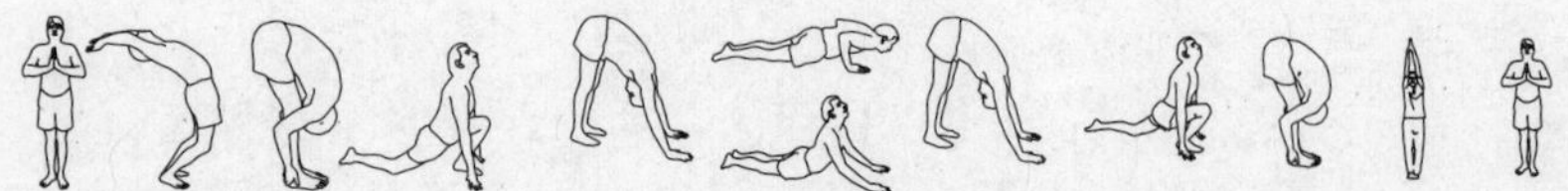

responses as compared to yoga trainees. A significant reduction in perceived exertion after maximal exercise in the yoga group after four to five months of yogic training was observed, which demonstrated the potential of yogic exercises in sports training and in different occupational situations both in the military and civil sectors. The data on oxidative stress recorded before and after exercise indicated that the subjects practising yogic exercises could successfully cope with oxidative stress by changes in three systems: increased metabolism of glutathione; elevated production of antioxidant enzymes; and more efficient elimination of per-oxidation products. Extensive research has also been carried out to examine the effect of yoga on neuro-physiological, hormonal and metabolic parameters. Erik Hoffman has tried to map the brain's activity after Kriya Yoga and found that following the meditation, a significant rise of alpha and theta rhythms in the brain was observed in ten out of eleven subjects. For some, the alpha waves more than doubled. The increase in these rhythms

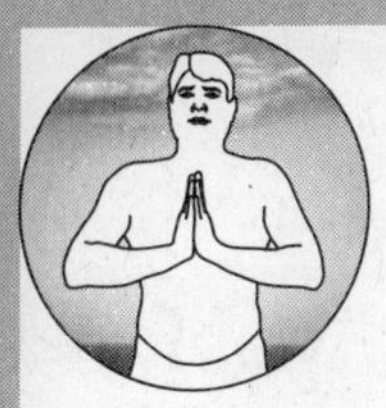

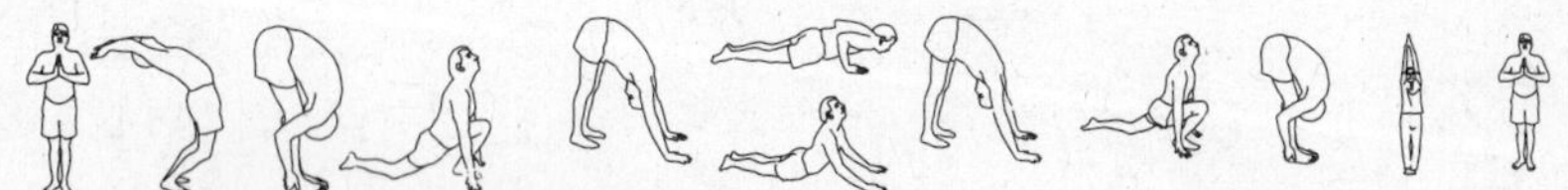

was greatest in the rear of the brain (parietal regions), where both alpha and theta rhythms rose by an average of forty per cent. There was a general tendency for these rhythms to spread from the rear of the brain to the front. In ten of the eleven right-handed people, the alpha increased more in the right than in the left side of the temporal regions. "The considerable increase in alpha and theta activity in most regions of the brain after meditation indicates that the brain is deeply relaxed and focused following Kriya Yoga. It also shows that through the meditation, the subjects have obtained a better contact with their subconscious and their emotions." The great increase of alpha rhythm in the right temporal lobe is an interesting finding. Recent research in the US has shown that depressed, introverted people have more alpha rhythm in the left fronto-temporal region, while optimistic, extrovert people have more in the right side. According to the American research, an increase of alpha rhythm in the right side, as found in this study of Kriya Yoga, counteracts

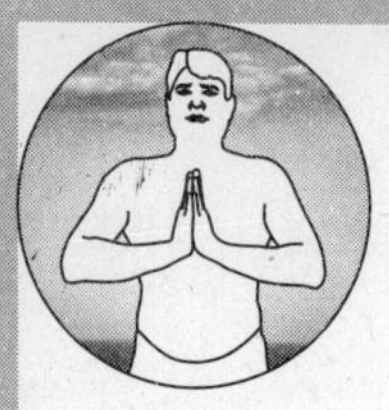

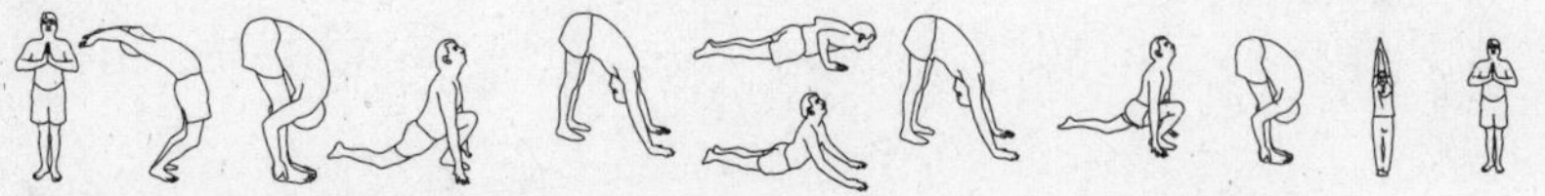

stress and depression. "Several scientific studies have demonstrated that theta rhythms in the EEG (mixed with alpha) correlate with the appearance of previously unconscious feelings, images and memories. Brain researchers claim that a person in the high alpha/theta state is able to confront and integrate unconscious processes."

Exercise-associated mood alterations have also been a subject of interest for the neurobiologists. It has been observed that people who perform yoga on a regular basis are in a better position to cope with stress as compared to people who do not. La Forge, Ralph (1995) have tried to delineate the mechanisms involved. Nearly all of us agree that exercise reduces tension and improves mental health; however, a specific cause-and-effect phenomenon has not been found. More than five decades of research has revealed numerous plausible mechanisms underlying exercise-related mood alterations. The review has revealed

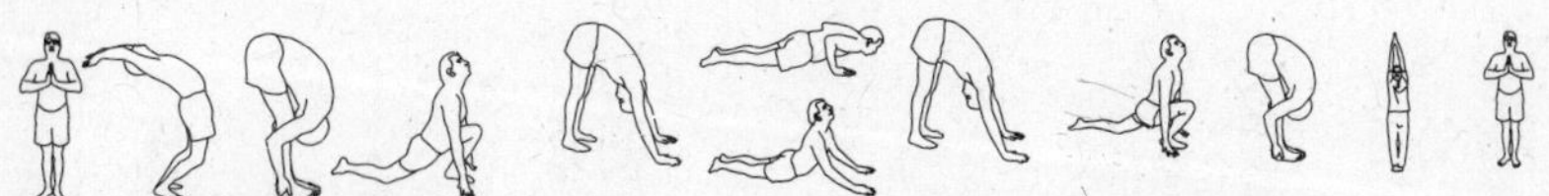

six of the more popular mechanisms which are often brought forward to explain the alterations of mood. Nearly all the mechanisms proposed, overlap or share some common neuro-anatomic pathway. It is probable that the best candidate for exercise-induced effective changes evolves from an integration of brain neurotransmission processes involving such principal neuroactive substances as endorphin, enkephalin, serotonin, dopamine and norepinephrine, among many others. The alliance of these specialised brain systems responsible for mood changes also influences a constellation of "mind-body" functions such as state-dependent learning and memory, autogenic training, eating behaviour, hypnosuggestion, psycho-neuro-immunology, and stress-related disorders such as hypertension. The utilisation of new brain imaging techniques to study acute exercise and collaborative efforts with researchers in cognitive neuroscience and neurobiology can help elucidate how these mechanisms are functionally coupled.

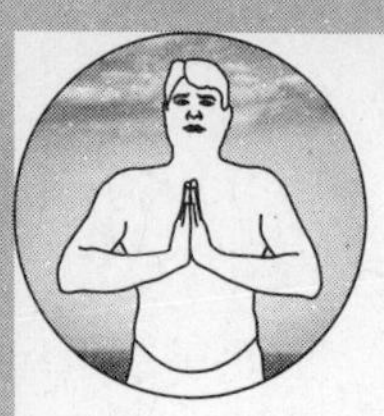

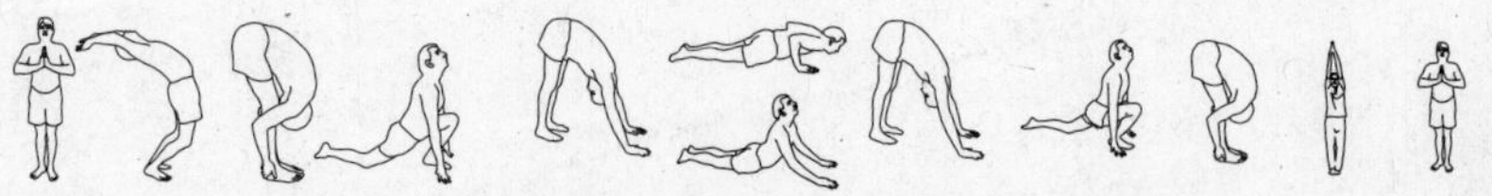

Individual psychobiological responses to exercise and other stimuli are invariably related to one's genetic code, the nature of the exercise, the exercise environment, and present health and fitness. By attempting to comprehend these extraordinary psychobiological features, fitness and health promotion professionals can better understand and respect individual differences in mood and performance. F.J. Schell (1994) measured heart rate, blood pressure, the hormones cortisol, prolactin and growth hormone and certain psychological parameters in a yoga practising group and a control group of young female volunteers reading in a comfortable position during the experimental period. There were no substantial differences between the groups concerning endocrine parameters and blood pressure. The course of heart rate was significantly different; the yoga group had a decrease during the yoga practice. Significant differences between both groups were found in psychological parameters. In the personality inventory the yoga group showed markedly higher scores

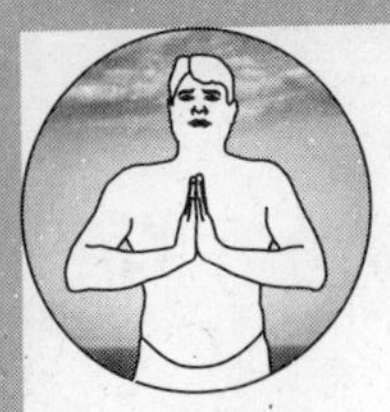

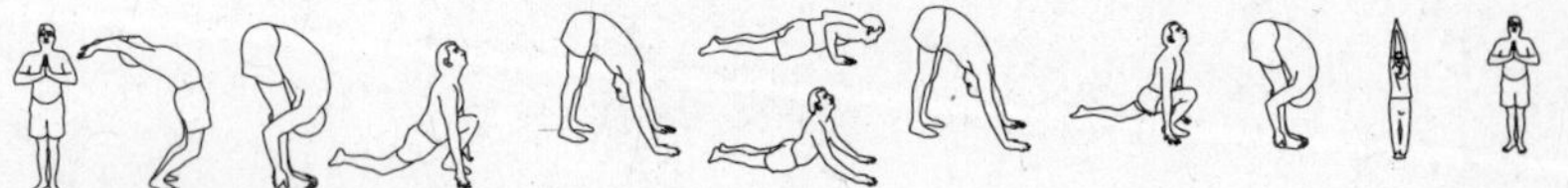

in life satisfaction and lower scores in excitability, aggressiveness, openness, emotionality and somatic complaints. Significant differences could also be observed concerning coping with stress and mood at the end of the experiment. The yoga group had significantly higher scores for high spirits and being extrovert.

Surya Namaskar is the combination of spinal bends, and the head is often kept at different heights in different positions. Some studies have tried to reveal the possible impact of the positions which keep the head at different levels on physiology. D. Konar *et al.* (2000) have tried to define the cardiovascular responses to the head-down-body-up postural exercise (Sarvangasana), which is a head-down-body-up postural exercise in a 'negative g' condition. This paper reports the results of the first systematic investigation on SVGN employing echocardiographic analysis in eight healthy male subjects before and after a practice of this asana twice daily for two weeks. The resting heart rate (HR) and left ventricular end

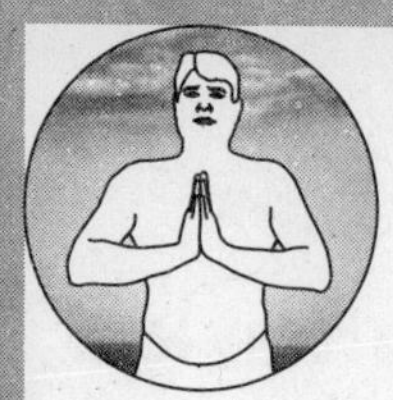

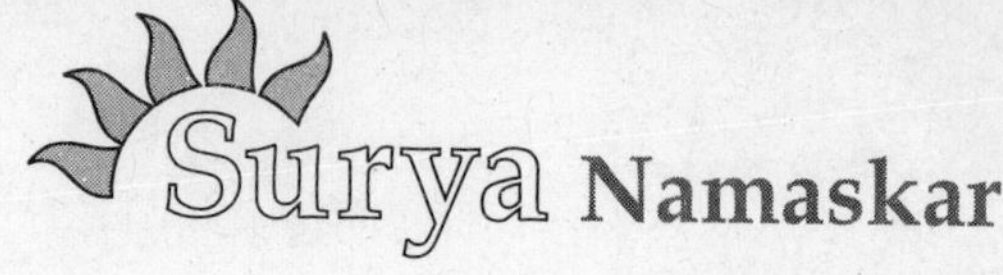

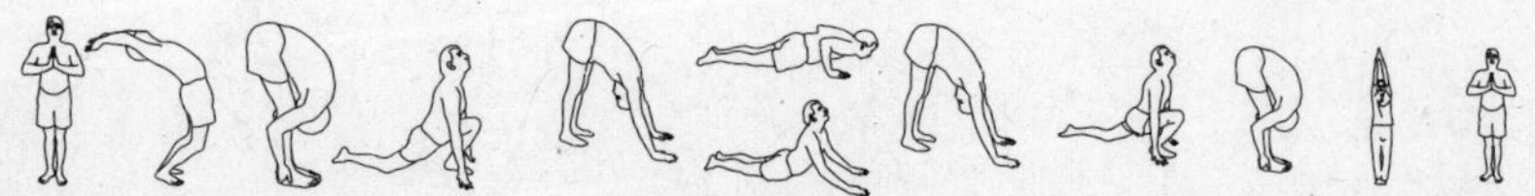

diastolic volume (LVEDV) were significantly reduced after practising this asana. A tendency towards a mild regression of the left ventricular mass was noticed, though it was not statistically significant. The CV responses to acute 45 degrees head-down tilt (HDT) in a tilt table was not altered after practising this asana. Also, there was no orthostatic intolerance during the 3-5 minute period of 70 degrees head-up tilt (HUT). These results strongly indicated that further studies of this asana performed for a longer period is likely to yield significant observations of applied value.

Forward bends—the structural and functional physiology

Spinal bending not only causes impacts upon the stretching spine but has a dynamic effect upon every part of the body involved directly or indirectly. Some of the impacts on different tissues and organs can be postulated as follows :

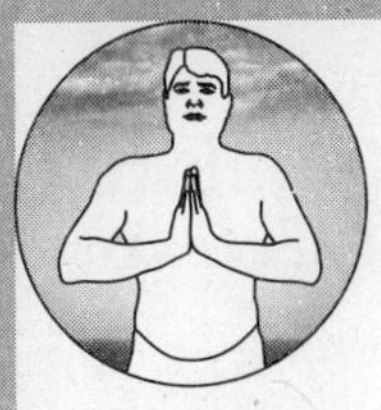

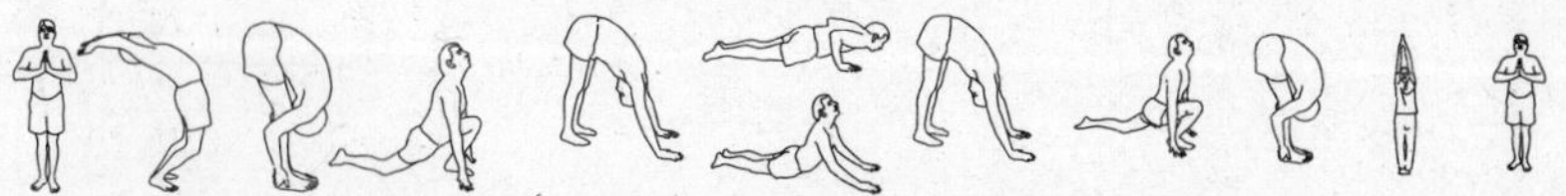

Physical : Hips are kept in dog tilt; vertebrae permit up to 90 degree flexion. Stretches entire back of body, especially legs and lower back. Elongates the spine outwards through the crown of your head as you fold into the pose. Movement from the hips and not the waist create movement/stronger pressure on the abdomen region, giving a massage effect and allowing for greater flexion of the spine.

Muscles : Legs, buttocks, abdomen, thorax spine, back and neck. Stretches the hamstrings, calves, and hips. Strengthens the thighs and knees. Prompts the spine to be in its natural position which, in general, is lost through the bad posture of a Western lifestyle. Extends the vertebrae allowing them to separate, thus stimulating the nerves to improve circulation in the spine, nourishing the cord.

Physiology : Compressor and massage to the abdominal organs, liver, kidneys, pancreas and intestines. Improved blood flow along the spine – oxygen to the brain.

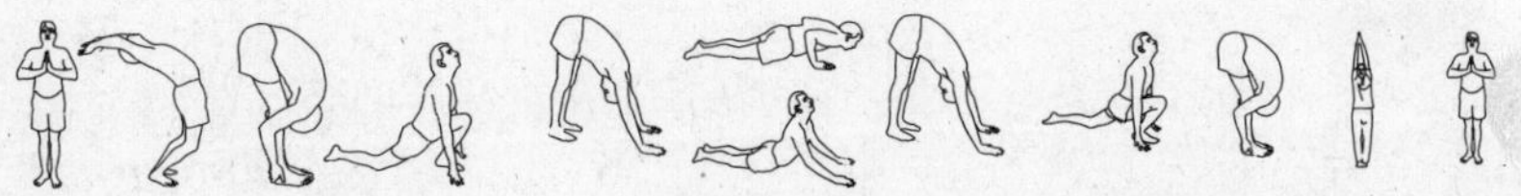

Improves digestion. Helps relieve the symptoms of menopause. Parasympathetic, encourages the relaxation response, lowering head and blood pressure.

Organs : Massages internal organs, tones liver, spleen, kidneys. Increases blood circulation to legs, torso, and brain. Tones spinal nerves asana for compressing the pelvis and the vata region.

Glands : Forward bends work on the first of the glands – the gonads or sex glands. Creativity and sex – the creative power posture – works on the endocrine glands. Forward bends and twists also quieten the adrenals. The upper back, kidneys, and adrenaline glands are stretched and stimulated, thus making forward bends a potentially therapeutic pose for those with respiratory or kidney problems, as well as for those who suffer from adrenal exhaustion.

Backward Bends – Anatomy and Physiology

Backbends are particularly strengthening for the

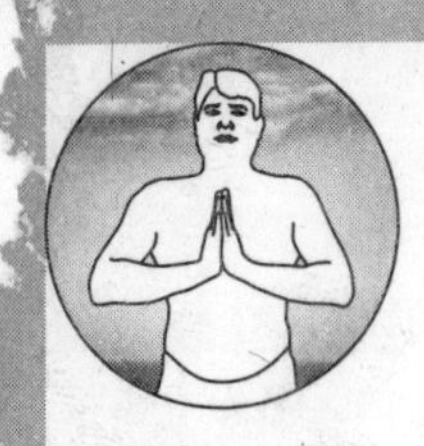

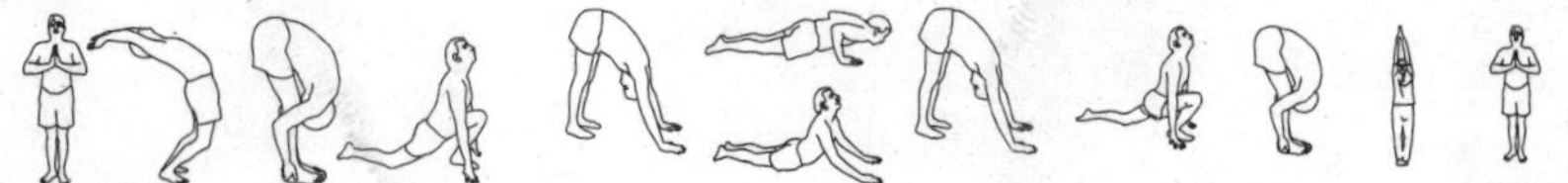

muscles that cause spinal extension - the erector spinae and the smaller semispinalis, multifidus and rotatores muscles that connect the bony processes of individual vertebrae. The muscles at the front of the body are stretched - psoas and illiacus muscles (hip flexors), the quadriceps muscle (hip and leg flexors) and the rectus abdominus muscles in the abdomen. The triceps muscles of the upper arms are strengthened and the intercostal muscles and pectoralis major are stretched.

Physiologically the endocrine glands in front of the body are stimulated - the pancreas which secretes hormones for carbohydrate metabolism, the thymus which regulates the immune function and the adrenals which influence our general state of alertness and arousal. The muscular activity produces heat and increased circulation. The opening of the chest improves the capacity of the lungs to expand on inhalation. The sympathetic nervous system is stimulated.

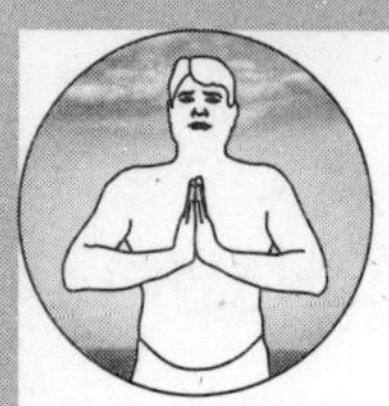

Surya Namaskar

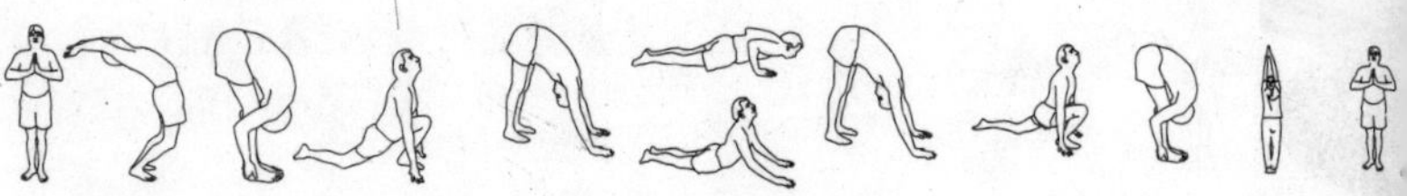

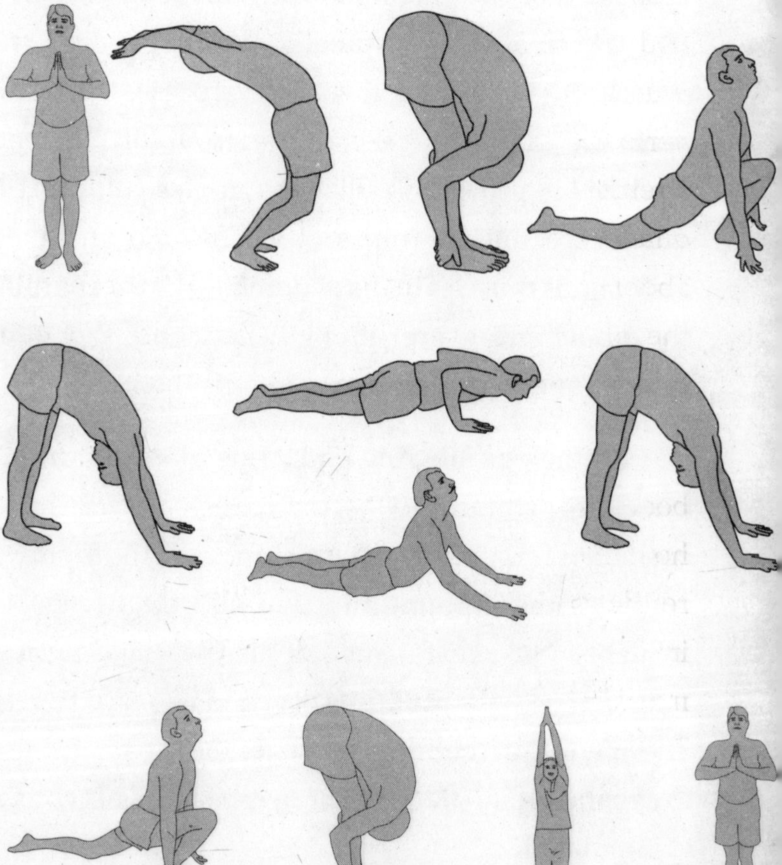

Complete Cycle of Surya Namaskar

8. Suggested Readings

1. *The Worship of Nature* — **James G. Frazer, 1925**
2. *The Two Republics* — **A.T. Jones**
3. *Surya Namaskar dwara Prakritik Swasthaya* — **Neelam Kumar, 1997**
4. *Vaidik Vangmaya me Prakritika Chikitsa* — **Ananta Bharati, 2004**
5. *Adi Urja Prana* — **Amrita Bharati, 2002**
6. *Yoga the Science of Love* — **Rajanish**
7. *Solar UV radiation effect on biological systems from physics in medicine and biology 36(3): 299-328 by Diffey BL1991*
8. *The Foundation of Contemporary Yoga* — **R.H. Singh 1991**
9. *Yogik Chikitsa* — **Swami Kuvalayananda, 1971**
10. *Swasthya ke liye Yoga* — **Sadashiva Nimbalkar, 1997**
11. *Light on Yoga* — **BKS Iyengar, 1976**

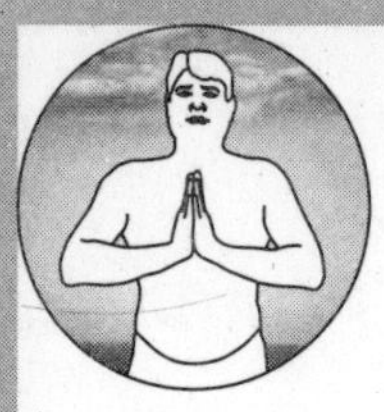

12. *Seminar on Yoga, Science and Man* **CCRIM&H** **1975**

13. *Psycho-physiological Effects of Yoga* **Trisha lamb** **2004**

14. *Yoga and Healing – Scientific Connections* **A.K. Malhotra** **2005**

15. Konar, D.R. Latha, and J.S. Bhuvaneswaran. Cardiovascular responses to head-down-body-up postural exercise (*Sarvangasana*). *Indian Journal of Physiology and Pharmacology*, October 2000, 44(4):392-400. PMID: 11214493.

16. Ramamurthi, B. Yoga and brain mechanisms with special reference to inhibitions. *The Yoga Review*, Summer 1982, 2(2):61-67.

17. La Forge, Ralph. Exercise-associated mood alterations: Interactive neurobiologic mechanisms. *Medicine, Exercise, Nutrition and Health*, 1995, 4:17-32.

18. Schell, F. J., B. Allolio, and O. W. Schonecke. Physiological and psychological effects of Hatha-Yoga exercise in healthy women. *International Journal of Psychosomatics*, 1994, 41(1-4):46-52.

□□□